Santal Women and the Health Care Regime

Faraha Nawaz • AN Bushra

Santal Women and the Health Care Regime

Pandemic, Predicament and Access

palgrave
macmillan

Faraha Nawaz
Department of Public Administration
University of Rajshahi
Rajshahi, Bangladesh

AN Bushra
Department of Public Administration
University of Rajshahi
Rajshahi, Bangladesh

ISBN 978-3-031-48871-9   ISBN 978-3-031-48872-6   (eBook)
https://doi.org/10.1007/978-3-031-48872-6

This Palgrave Macmillan imprint is published by the registered company Springer Nature Switzerland AG.
The registered company address is: Gewerbestrasse 11, 6330 Cham, Switzerland

Paper in this product is recyclable.

A Glimpse Ahead

In the annals of human history, moments arise that demand our collective attention, challenging us to confront our biases, address systemic inequalities, and reevaluate the fundamental principles that underpin our societies. The COVID-19 pandemic stands as one such epochal juncture, laying bare the vulnerabilities and disparities that persist within our global healthcare systems. Within this tumultuous landscape, the experiences of marginalized communities, often relegated to the periphery of mainstream discourse, emerge as poignant narratives that compel us to critically reflect on the state of healthcare access and equity.

This book delves into the intricate tapestry of healthcare access for Santal women during the unprecedented challenges posed by the COVID-19 pandemic. The Santal community, an indigenous population inhabiting the Northern regions of Bangladesh and neighboring countries, has historically grappled with multifaceted socio-economic and cultural disparities. The pandemic, with its far-reaching implications, has acted as a crucible, intensifying pre-existing vulnerabilities and casting a glaring light on the entrenched barriers that hinder their access to essential healthcare services.

Based on thorough research, personal accounts, and a range of perspectives from different fields, this book strives to untangle the intricate connections among gender, ethnicity, socio-economic influences, and healthcare availability within the framework of the Santal community. It sheds light on the myriad challenges faced by Santal women—challenges often exacerbated by traditional healthcare practices, limitations of the healthcare delivery system, multiple identity factors, and inadequate resources. These obstacles, magnified in the wake of COVID-19, serve as a stark reminder of the urgent need for a more inclusive and equitable healthcare system that leaves no one behind.

Through the pages of this book, we immerse ourselves in the lived experiences of Santal women—about the problems they faced and the way they tried to stay strong. In doing so, we confront uncomfortable truths and confront the deeply ingrained disparities that have persisted for generations. But within these narratives of adversity, we also find stories of resilience, adaptation to the new normal, and the unwavering determination to overcome adversity and to change their fate. As we navigate the intricate narrative threads woven throughout this exploration, we are beckoned to reevaluate our understanding of healthcare as a universal right. The Santal women's journey through the COVID-19 pandemic calls on us to challenge the status quo, advocate for transformative change, and foster an environment where healthcare is not merely a privilege, but a fundamental pillar of human dignity.

This book stands as a testament to the societal discrimination against Santal women in their pursuit of health, equality, and justice. It is an invitation to engage with their stories, confront the structural inequities that persist, and collectively forge a path toward a more just and inclusive future. May this book inspire discourse, spark activism, and ignite the flames of change as we strive to ensure that the lessons learned from this pandemic lead us to a world where healthcare access is a reality for all, regardless of gender, ethnicity, or circumstance.

ACKNOWLEDGMENTS

Writing this book on the healthcare access of Santal women during the COVID-19 pandemic has been a collaborative effort that would not have been possible without the support, guidance, and contributions of numerous individuals and organizations. We extend our heartfelt gratitude to all those who have played a pivotal role in making this endeavor a reality.

First and foremost, we express our deepest appreciation to the Santal women, their family members, and their community leaders who generously shared their experiences, insights, and stories with us. Their resilience, struggle, and strength in the face of challenges have been a constant source of inspiration, and this book stands as a testament to their voices and struggles. We would also like to acknowledge the contribution made by the officials of DASCOH Foundation who sacrificed their valuable time for us during our field study.

Our sincere thanks go to the healthcare professionals, community leaders, and advocates who participated in interviews, discussions, and surveys, providing invaluable perspectives and information that enriched the content of this book. We would like to extend our sincere thanks to the healthcare providers of the NUHC, especially Dr. Sultana Papia, who has given me the time to interview her from her very busy schedule. We are also grateful to Rehana Khatun Tultuli, former vice chairman of Nachol Upazila Parishad, who helped us a lot to communicate with the officials of Upazila Health Complex Nachol and guided us in the field visits. Without her connections and guidance, data collection for this study would have been very difficult.

We are also thankful to Ataelahi Usama for his continuous support and company in the field visits, recording the interviews, and taking pictures during the field visits. And lastly, we are indebted to our families for their unwavering encouragement and understanding throughout the journey of researching and writing this book. Your patience and support provided us with the necessary foundation to delve into this crucial topic.

We extend our appreciation to the reviewers and editors who contributed their expertise to refine the manuscript and enhance its readability and academic rigor. Last but not least, we recognize the readers of this book, who will engage with the knowledge and insights presented herein. Your interest and engagement contribute to the ongoing dialogue surrounding healthcare access, gender disparities, and the impact of the pandemic.

CONTENTS

1 Preface   1

2 Equality and Inclusivity in the Healthcare System of
  Bangladesh   25

3 Healthcare Access and Ethnic Women's Right to Health:
  A Void in the Literature   37

4 Healthcare on the Margins: Santal Women's Access
  Through an Intersectional Lens   51

5 Unveiling Santal Women's Healthcare Challenges During
  the Pandemic   71

6 Unlocking New Perspectives: Lessons and Future Avenues   93

Index   109

LIST OF FIGURES

Fig. 1.1   Map of Nachol Upazila. (Source: Bangladesh National
           Portal, n.d.)   14
Fig. 1.2   Hakroil village in photos   15
Fig. 1.3   Lakkhanpur village in photos   17
Fig. 2.1   The healthcare system of Bangladesh. (Source: Adapted from
           Masud Ahmed et al., 2015)   29
Fig. 2.2   Different levels of public healthcare services in Bangladesh.
           (Source: Adapted from DGHS, 2022)   30
Fig. 3.1   Levesque's conceptual framework of access to health. (Source:
           Levesque et al., 2013)   39
Fig. 3.2   Andersen's healthcare utilization model. (Source: Andersen,
           1995, p. 8)   41
Fig. 3.3   Intersectional framework to study access to healthcare. (Source:
           Authors)   43
Fig. 4.1   COVID-19 awareness-building posters in Santal villages by
           DASCOH foundation   64
Fig. 4.2   COVID-19 vaccination awareness efforts by DASCOH
           foundation   65
Fig. 4.3   COVID-19 vaccination corner at the NUHC   67

LIST OF TABLES

Table 1.1   The five dimensions of accessibility by Levesque et al. (2013)   12
Table 1.2   Five dimensions of accessibility by Penchansky and Thomas   13
Table 4.1   Santal women's frequency of visiting healthcare facilities
during COVID-19   52
Table 4.2   Frequency of seeking healthcare across gender and ethnic
groups during COVID-19   56
Table 4.3   Average level of education of the respondents   59
Table 4.4   COVID-19-induced behavioral change   62
Table 4.5   Vaccination rate of the respondents   66
Table 5.1   Major reasons for not choosing UHC as a healthcare
destination   72
Table 5.2   Changed financial status during COVID-19   79
Table 5.3   Santal women's sources of healthcare financing   81
Table 5.4   Factors limiting Santal women's access to telemedicine service   87

CHAPTER 1

Preface

Abstract Gender and class inequality are pervasive in Bangladesh. This inequality is gravely felt by those who belong to multiple marginalized social categories such as ethnic women, who are subject to social marginalization due to their gender and ethnic identity. The majority of the ethnic women in rural Bangladesh live in obsequious poverty, having very poor access to various types of public services including healthcare. Neither the government nor the market initiatives have been successful in addressing the healthcare needs of ethnic women, especially those living in the north of Bangladesh, including the Santal women. The overall accessibility to healthcare of the Santal women deteriorated as a global pandemic broke out in 2019. This chapter analyzes the prioritization of equal and equitable healthcare for all by various international treaties and health policies of the Government of Bangladesh (GoB) and the status of Santal women's access to healthcare. Some key concepts of the research have been described in this chapter for a better understanding of the core concepts of the book. This chapter also presents an overview of the research design adopted for this research. The chapter provides justification for the choice of research frame, research sites, methods, and the overall research process.

Keywords Intersectionality • Access • Public health • COVID-19 • Santal women

This book is a case study of Santal women's access to healthcare during the COVID-19 pandemic in Bangladesh. It examines the extent of healthcare accessibility of ethnic women from the Santal tribe and the role of intersectional identity in their healthcare accessibility in Bangladesh, as well as the challenges limiting their healthcare access during a global pandemic. The book begins with the background of equal healthcare rights in the context of the healthcare policies of Bangladesh and the existing discrimination in the healthcare system so that the reader can understand the importance of writing a book on this topic.

Health is a key indicator of human development. It is fundamental for improving the Quality of Life (QoL) of people. Improved health is a precondition for national development, as better health has a positive influence on income, education, and the overall well-being of the people. Considering its immense importance, the right to health has been preserved in a number of human rights treaties, international organizations, and national constitutions around the world, for instance, the Constitution of the World Health Organization (WHO) (1946), Article 251 of the Universal Declaration of Human Rights (1948), and Article 12 of the International Covenant on Economic, Social, and Cultural Rights (1966). The right to health is recognized by all states in the world as each state has ratified at least one international human rights treaty that has provisions to acknowledge the right to health (UNHCHR, 2008).

The Constitution of the People's Republic of Bangladesh has recognized healthcare as a fundamental need and prioritized the state's role in ensuring primary healthcare for its citizens. Under the domain of the Fundamental Principles of State Policy, Article 15(a), Article 16, and Article 18 of the Constitution are mentioned here. According to Article 15(a), the provision of medical care along with other basic necessities, including food, clothing, shelter, and education, shall be a fundamental responsibility of the State. Article 16 has emphasized the development of public health in rural areas and removing disparities in living standards between rural and urban areas. Article 18(1) is probably the most important provision regarding public health, as it specifies the provision of public healthcare as a primary role of the state.

Although the legal basis for equitable healthcare provision is quite strong in both global and Bangladeshi contexts, its applicability is subject to various socio-political and cultural factors, as evidence suggests that not all social groups enjoy equal access to healthcare and that the implementation of a health policy produces different outcomes for different social groups. Some groups always have better access than others. Also, although these provisions of international treaties and national constitutions provide a base for equal healthcare for all in normal situations, the mechanisms to address abnormal situations like a global pandemic are still inadequate and inefficient (Hannon et al., 2022). Existing studies suggest that women, subject to different disadvantaged social groups, have experienced the pandemic and its effect on healthcare access at varying intensities (Chowdhury et al., 2022; Behar, 2020; Ryan & El Ayadi, 2020; Ellington et al., 2020; Akhtar, 2020).

Despite the existing studies, there is a serious inadequacy of research in the South Asian context that has adopted an intersectional approach to identify within-group inequalities experienced by women from different ethnic, disadvantaged, and vulnerable social groups. This inadequacy has led to the emergence of a lack of evidence and a lack of awareness of the healthcare needs of women. Ignoring the dynamic aspect of inequality only leads to institutionalizing and establishing inequality as a common social norm. Thus, taking a comprehensive approach to addressing inequality is fundamental to removing oppression and injustice toward certain communities. The current study aims to investigate the experiences of Santal women in accessing healthcare services during the COVID-19 pandemic in order to differentiate their experiences based on various identity markers and factors of disadvantage. By doing so, the present study will address the existing gap in the academic literature.

HEALTHCARE ACCESSIBILITY IN THE NEW NORMAL

The COVID-19 pandemic, caused by the novel coronavirus SARS-CoV-2, has had far-reaching impacts on countries around the world, including Bangladesh. This South Asian nation, with a population exceeding 160 million people, faced unique challenges and experiences throughout the course of the pandemic. In this chapter, we will delve into the COVID-19 situation in Bangladesh, spanning from the initial outbreak to the evolving response measures and societal implications. The journey of Bangladesh through the COVID-19 pandemic began in early 2020 when the virus was first detected within its borders. Like many countries, Bangladesh faced a daunting task: to protect its population from the highly contagious virus while grappling with limited healthcare resources. In the initial phase, the government swiftly implemented strict lockdown measures, closing schools and businesses, and restricting movement to contain the virus's spread (Dhaka Tribune, 2020). However, the healthcare system faced significant challenges such as a shortage of testing facilities and difficulties in contact tracing. Hospitals were often overwhelmed as they struggled to accommodate a growing number of COVID-19 patients, revealing vulnerabilities that had long existed within the healthcare infrastructure.

As time progressed, Bangladesh made strides in its response efforts. Testing and contact tracing capabilities were improved, allowing for more effective identification and isolation of cases. International aid and support played a pivotal role in bolstering the healthcare system, providing critical medical supplies, and strengthening the capacity of healthcare workers. Additionally, multiple COVID-19 vaccines were approved for emergency use, providing hope for eventual control over the virus. However, challenges persisted, including vaccine supply issues and vaccine hesitancy among certain segments of the population. This hesitancy can be addressed through clear, accessible, and tailored information campaigns. However, stigma, discrimination, limited access to quality healthcare, and distrust in the government exacerbate these issues and distance these populations from public health services (Ullah & Chattoraj, 2022). The healthcare system, especially in densely populated urban areas and in remote rural villages, faced immense pressure. Reports of shortages of hospital beds, oxygen, and other essential medical supplies emerged in some regions. To curb the virus's spread, authorities implemented intermittent lockdowns and restrictions, which, while necessary, had socio-economic consequences (The Daily Star, 2021).

During the outbreak of COVID-19, 219 countries, territories, and areas put into effect an astounding 60,711 pandemic-related restrictions, resulting in unparalleled historical actions. These measures encompassed severe steps such as border closures, quarantines, expulsions, and lockdowns, specifically aimed at migrants, refugees, and displaced populations (Ullah et al., 2021). Chapainawabganj, a border district in Bangladesh, faced significant vulnerabilities during the COVID-19 pandemic, primarily due to its proximity to India and the emergence of the deadly variant (Haque, 2021). The porous border allowed for the easy movement of people and goods, making it challenging to control the virus's spread (Abdullah, 2022). Limited healthcare infrastructure was a critical vulnerability as the sudden influx of COVID-19 cases strained resources, leading to shortages of hospital beds and medical supplies (Al-Zaman, 2020). Socio-economic factors, including a heavy reliance on agriculture and informal labor, exacerbated the district's vulnerability, with lockdowns disrupting livelihoods. Informal cross-border trade, essential for the local economy, became a potential avenue for the virus to spread due to limited testing and health screening.

The outbreak of the COVID-19 virus has had immense negative effects on public health and health service delivery, as well as on socio-political institutions and social harmony. Violence and inequality have grown as a result of prolonged lockdowns, economic division of society has reached its peak due to the layoffs that resulted at the beginning stage of the pandemic from the virus outbreak (Aziz et al., 2020; Kumar & Pinky, 2021), and the weaknesses of the existing healthcare system have come to light from the news reports on corruption, mismanagement of public funds, lack of coordination, and inefficiency in public healthcare facilities making the headlines of national dailies on a regular basis (Foyez, 2021). Two fundamental problems have massively grown during the pandemic but remained less explored by researchers and policymakers despite their grave intensity. As a result of prolonged lockdowns and the laying off of employees and workers, two rising issues that demand much attention are the problem of accessibility to public services and the growing inequality in society. The availability of a service alone is not very helpful unless the people who are meant to use it can access it. Growing inequality in terms of economic solvency and social class can lead to fragmentation of the society, paving the way for a chaotic environment for the policymakers to deal with existing problems.

Mandatory social distancing measures and lockdowns imposed by the government made it harder for rural people to access primary health services, let alone COVID-19-related healthcare, from the local government healthcare facilities. Upazila Health Complex (hereinafter UHC) is the first referral health facility at the primary level of the healthcare delivery system in Bangladesh. The UHCs provide treatment for the cases referred from the union level and also refer them to the district/ medical college hospitals when necessary. Upazila Health Complexes (along with Union Health and Family Welfare Centers) provide health and family planning services (Islam et al., 2019). Women and children are significant stakeholders in these facilities. However, studies revealed that females (53.3%) have poorer accessibility to the services of UHC than males (41.1%) (Islam et al., 2019). Another study has found that male patients are more content with the health services of UHC than female patients (Rumi et al., 2021). This poor accessibility and discontentment among female service recipients point to the unequal attitudes and practices that have long existed in the public service delivery system.

When a person falls into more than one disadvantaged category based on different identity determinants, they experience inequality and marginalization in a more severe form. When three identity markers (gender, poverty, and lack of education) come together, intersect, and form an identity in conjunction with each other, the intersecting elements of disadvantage scale up the vulnerability factors of the subject immensely. Thus, the level of inequality experienced by a poor Santal woman is much more different, complex, and severe than what a poor woman belonging to a non-ethnic group experiences. By studying the health behavior of the Santal women and the challenges of their healthcare accessibility resulting from their intersectional identity and the COVID-19 pandemic outbreak, this study is set to analyze the behavioral change and influence of the pandemic over factors of the Santal women's healthcare accessibility. And finally, this study attempts to identify how and to what extent the intersectional identity factors of Santal women have influenced their access to healthcare during the coronavirus pandemic.

This study adds value to the existing body of knowledge as well as provides a baseline for future researchers interested in exploring social change, access to public service during a health crisis, and intersectional analysis of inequality in the public service delivery systems in Bangladesh. This study can also be helpful to policymakers in realizing the real-life scenario of health-related policy implementation. This study can empower policy stakeholders with a better understanding of the marginalized and disadvantaged strata, which can improve the formulation and implementation of inclusive health policies in the future.

Women's Healthcare
from an Intersectional Perspective

Although the legal basis for equitable healthcare provision is quite strong in both global and Bangladeshi contexts, its applicability is subject to various socio-political and cultural factors, as evidence suggests that not all social groups enjoy equal access to healthcare and that the implementation of health policy produces different outcomes for different social groups. Some groups always have better access than others. The COVID-19 crisis has had distinct impacts on women and men, with women bearing a greater burden due to the pre-existing disparities in social, economic, and political domains (George & Kuruvilla, 2021). Also, although these provisions of international treaties and national constitutions provide a base for equal healthcare for all in normal situations, the mechanisms to address abnormal situations like a global pandemic are still inadequate and inefficient (Hannon et al., 2022). This inefficiency primarily stems from fragmented crisis management approaches, a focus on reacting rather than preventing, inadequate disaster preparedness, and a lack of coordination between healthcare systems and other sectors (WHO, 2019b).

Health emergency management–related plans and initiatives during COVID-19 were primarily focused on, but not limited to, the prevention and mitigation of health-related challenges. Globally, efforts by the states, non-governmental actors, and private organizations were directed toward dealing with the emerging social changes initiated by the pandemic along with the health hazards. Existing studies show growing concerns about the issues of education, unemployment, economic instability, social inequality, domestic violence and abuse, gender gap, and economic division, which are a resultant change of the pandemic (Islam & Hossain, 2021; Nicola et al., 2020; Rasul et al., 2021). Much of the COVID-19-related study conducted from a gender perspective has captured data related to vaccine hesitancy, the comparison of hospitalization ratios and death rates between men and women, and gender-based violence. Other sex and gender disaggregated data were not collected, monitored, and reported properly on a regular basis due to a lack of knowledge, resources, or political will (Morgan et al., 2022).

Women are the frontline workers of health service delivery across the globe, as 70% of the global health and social care workforce are women, who were the most exposed and vulnerable to the pandemic (WHO, 2019a). But studies reveal that the majority of healthcare workers who have died during this COVID-19 pandemic were women of color, who were subject to more than one vulnerable identity. One report reveals that in the USA, nurses of Filipino descent account for a shocking 31.5% of the workforce's COVID-19 deaths, although they make up only 4% of the workforce (Akhtar, 2020). The focus on the fact that more men are affected by and die from the virus tends to overlook the role of gender-related social factors in the spread of the virus and the differences in vulnerability within specific groups of people.

Poor, ethnic, and disabled women had lower access to support in abusive relationships during COVID-19 than women who were financially solvent, non-ethnic, and able-bodied (Ryan & El Ayadi, 2020). Other data from the USA shows that Hispanic and non-Hispanic Black pregnant women were affected disproportionately by COVID-19 infection during pregnancy, as they experienced an increased hospitalization rate, a higher rate of admission to the ICU, and received mechanical ventilation (Ellington et al., 2020). Gender data for different women's groups in Latin America during COVID-19 wasn't found. However, in Latin America, during the Zika epidemic of 2015–2017, indigenous women had poorer access to contraceptives than non-indigenous women (Darney et al., 2017).

Data on intersectional analysis of differential treatments and experiences of women in the context of South Asia and Bangladesh is scarce. However, some studies have attempted to discuss the inequality of treatment and outcome brought toward marginalized communities during the pandemic from an intersectional viewpoint (although not all of these studies have adopted intersectionality as the main theoretical framework for their studies). Behar (2020) reported that girls and women in India had experienced limited access to menstrual and hygiene products during COVID-19. The experiences of women living in urban, rural, and remote regions of this country significantly differed in this context. Citing data from the National Family and Health Survey–4 of India, she noted that only 26.4% of girls (of the age group of 15–24) living in the rural region and 65.4% of girls living in the urban region of India use absorbing material during their periods. Chowdhury et al. (2022), in their study, tried to capture the intersectional differential treatments experienced by disabled women in Bangladesh, along with other factors that enhance the disadvantages of disability.

Existing studies from global, South Asian, and Bangladeshi contexts suggest that women, subject to different disadvantaged social groups, have experienced the pandemic and its outcome with varying intensity. But there is a serious inadequacy of studies in the South Asian context that have adopted an intersectional approach to identify these within group inequalities experienced by women of different ethnic, disadvantaged, and marginalized social groups. Due to this, a lack of evidence and awareness of the healthcare needs of women have emerged. Ignoring the dynamic aspect of inequality only leads to the institutionalization and establishment of inequality as a common social norm. Thus, taking a comprehensive approach to addressing inequality is fundamental to removing oppression and injustice toward certain communities. The present study aims at exploring the experiences of rural ethnic women from the Santal tribe in accessing healthcare services during the COVID-19 pandemic outbreak and differentiating their experiences on the basis of a number of identity markers and factors of disadvantage. This study further examines the role of Santal patriarchy in producing systematic inequality and barriers for women in healthcare access. By doing so, the present study will address the existing gap in the academic literature.

Conceptual Perplexity: Public Health, Public Healthcare, and Public Healthcare Services

One of the key concepts in this book is public health. Public Health is an empirical and multidisciplinary field that aims to assure conditions in which people can be healthy. The underlying principle of public health is to deal with the health of the population in its totality by undertaking a precautionary measure rather than a responsive measure. Health interventions under public health include community hygiene, sanitation, health education, immunization, and nutrition promotion (Schmitt & Schmitt, 2008). This view of public health emphasizes the prevention of a disease and can be described as the avoidance of any health trouble that has the potential to affect the health and well-being of the mass public. In other words, public health is a set of precautionary steps that attempt to prevent disease and promote the collective health of a population. Public health is only concerned with common health issues that may affect the general well-being of a large population and not individual patients.

The term public health is often confused with the concept of 'public healthcare'. Public health, as described above, is concerned with precautionary health measures concerning the well-being of people and communities in general. Whereas public healthcare is a system by which the healthcare needs of a community are met. Healthcare involves the prevention, diagnosis, treatment, and curing of all types of physical and mental health problems in people by trained medical professionals. The fundamental difference between 'public health' and 'public healthcare' is that public health is only concerned with precautionary measures, whereas public healthcare is concerned with both precautionary and curative measures to address the healthcare needs of a population in general. Healthcare services, on the other hand, may include services related to prevention, treatment of a health hazard, or rehabilitation after experiencing a health risk (WHO, 2020).

The term 'public healthcare' is defined and used by researchers and public health professionals, by and large, from two perspectives. One group of experts defines public healthcare services as healthcare services provided by government-operated facilities and funded by public money. From this point of view, healthcare services can largely be divided into (1) public healthcare and (2) private healthcare (Mannan, 2013; Pallegedara & Grimm, 2017). Public healthcare are healthcare products and services provided by the government-run facilities and funded majorly by public money, whereas private healthcare is provided by facilities that are usually profit-making institutions and operated by private entities (Mannan, 2013; Pallegedara & Grimm, 2017). Private healthcare, on the contrary, is healthcare services provided by individuals and organizations that are neither owned nor directly controlled by governments. Private healthcare services can have any of the following forms: for profit and non-profit, formal and informal, and domestic and international (WHO, 2020).

The second perspective on public healthcare, as held by some researchers and practitioners, depicts it as healthcare services that are concerned only with public health irrespective of the nature of the providers. This happens when sometimes public healthcare is provided and managed by healthcare 'enterprises' or a comprehensive group of health service providers, including public, private, and voluntary organizations (Malakoane et al., 2020). Public healthcare services involve collaboration among various entities, including public, private, and voluntary institutions, working collectively to provide essential public health services to the population (CDC, 2021). This view incorporates elements of public health in the definition of 'public healthcare service' and excludes individual health concerns regardless of whether the treatment was received from a government-run facility or a privately owned hospital. In simpler words, public healthcare services, from the second point of view, are those healthcare services that deal with health issues affecting people and communities in general (COVID-19 vaccination, for instance) irrespective of the providers.

The first perspective on public healthcare examines it based on funding and provider characteristics, while the second viewpoint shifts focus away from providers and highlights the nature of health issues and their impact on a substantial portion of the population. This definition limits its focus on the government-run institutions to promote collective health and well-being. The second definition ensures the inclusion of both public and privately owned and run health facilities and healthcare providers in the provision of healthcare to a mass of people. Thus, the use of the term 'Public healthcare' incorporates both of its meanings. It can either be health services delivered through government-run and publicly funded facilities or any public, private, or voluntary institution that provides services to deal with public health–related problems.

Although public health is one aspect of public healthcare, confusion between the two terms is common in public discourse. The present study makes a distinction between public health, public healthcare, and public healthcare services. Public health aims to deal with the general health of the population in its totality by undertaking a precautionary measure rather than taking on a responsive measure. Public healthcare involves activities regarding the prevention, diagnosis, treatment, and curing of all types of physical and mental health problems of general people, often funded by public money and provided by the government. Healthcare services refer to medical services required for diagnosis and treatment of individual patients. So, the main point of disagreement between the two terms 'public health', and 'public healthcare', is in their nature and focus. Public health denotes purely precautionary actions; public healthcare is concerned with both precautionary and curative measures.

EXPLICATION OF ACCESSIBILITY IN HEALTHCARE LITERATURE

The term access to healthcare, as put forward by Gulliford et al. (2002), is concerned with the link between healthcare need, healthcare provision, and the utilization of health services. From this point of view, healthcare access and utilization revolve around the relationship between health service providers and service recipients. Gulliford et al. (2002) have further elaborated their view on access to healthcare, noting that the concept 'access' can be seen in two terms: in terms of having access and/or in terms of gaining access. Having access to a service means that the service in demand is available for use, and there is also a working system that allows the utilization of the service. On the other hand, gaining access refers to the actual procedure of getting into the processes of utilizing the service available. It denotes entry to, or utilization of, healthcare services (Gulliford et al., 2002).

Levesque et al. (2013) have conceptualized access by exploring five dimensions of it capturing both supply side and demand side determinants. The five dimensions of accessibility include (Table 1.1):

These five dimensions of accessibility are closely related to the five dimensions of ability of the service recipients which include ability to perceive, ability to seek, ability to reach, ability to pay, and ability to engage. These determinants are subject to ecological, financial, and organizational obstacles (Levesque et al., 2013).

Penchansky and Thomas (1981) (cited in Gulliford et al., 2002) suggested that the concept of access described the 'degree of fit' between clients and the health system. They identified five relevant dimensions to the client–service interaction (Table 1.2).

Access to healthcare in the existing literature has been conceptualized comprehensively. In this study, this concept is used to capture all the notions of this term as expressed above. In this study, access to healthcare refers to the affordability of healthcare services by the general public in terms of financial ability, favorable attitude of the service providers, adequate supply of healthcare products and services, availability of healthcare providers, physical and locational factors, and the ability to finally utilize the available healthcare services. In the assessment of access to healthcare services, the focus is given to public healthcare services, that is, health services provided by the government-run healthcare facilities. However, some supporting data regarding the contribution of private and

Table 1.1 The five dimensions of accessibility by Levesque et al. (2013)

Approachability	Identification by the patient of existing healthcare services that can be reached and that might have an impact on the health of the individual.
Acceptability	Cultural and social factors that determine the healthcare decision of a patient as in whether people would accept some aspects of the service (e.g. the sex or social group of providers) or not.
Availability and accommodation	Health services (in the form of the physical space or those working in healthcare roles) are reachable both physically and in a timely manner.
Affordability	The economic capacity of people to spend resources and time to access health services
Appropriateness	A match between available services and the need of the recipients, its timeliness, the amount of care spent, and the technical aspects and quality of the services.

Source: Adapted from Levesque et al. (2013, p. 5)

Table 1.2 Five dimensions of accessibility by Penchansky and Thomas

Acceptability	Attitudes of service recipients and service providers about each other's characteristics.
Affordability	The direct and indirect costs and the perceived value of the health service in relation to the needs of the patients.
Availability	Adequacy of supply against the types of services (provision) and type of needs (demand).
Physical accessibility	The location of the service in relation to the distance and mobility of the patient (geographical and physical barriers).
Accommodation	The way services are organized in relation to the client's needs (opening times, booking facilities, waiting times).

Source: Adapted from Penchansky and Thomas (1981) as cited in Gulliford et al. (2002, p. 19)

non-governmental agencies in the healthcare provision is also tracked and covered in this study.

THE RESEARCH TERRAIN

The initial research was conducted in Bangladesh through a pilot study in 2021. Then comprehensive research was conducted through a number of visits in 2022 and early 2023 from time to time. In each visit, rural ethnic women (from Santal tribe), their family members, village people, community leaders, NGO officials, local politicians, and healthcare providers at the Upazila Health Complex were communicated. The study was conducted in two villages: Hakroil village and Paschim Lakkhanpur village of Nachol Upazila, Chapainawabganj district, Bangladesh (Fig. 1.1).

Sociological Case-Study Design

To find answers to the research questions, a case-oriented qualitative research strategy is the best suited method for several reasons. Case-oriented studies are effective in studies that ask 'How' and 'Why' questions and the subjects of the study can relate to a real life context. In the collection and analysis of data, qualitative research strategy usually focuses more on textual descriptions and not on numerical data. Qualitative research is an appropriate method to pick when a study wishes to examine the 'human side' of an issue, which includes intangible elements like gender, socio-economic status, norms and values, ethnicity, and religion.

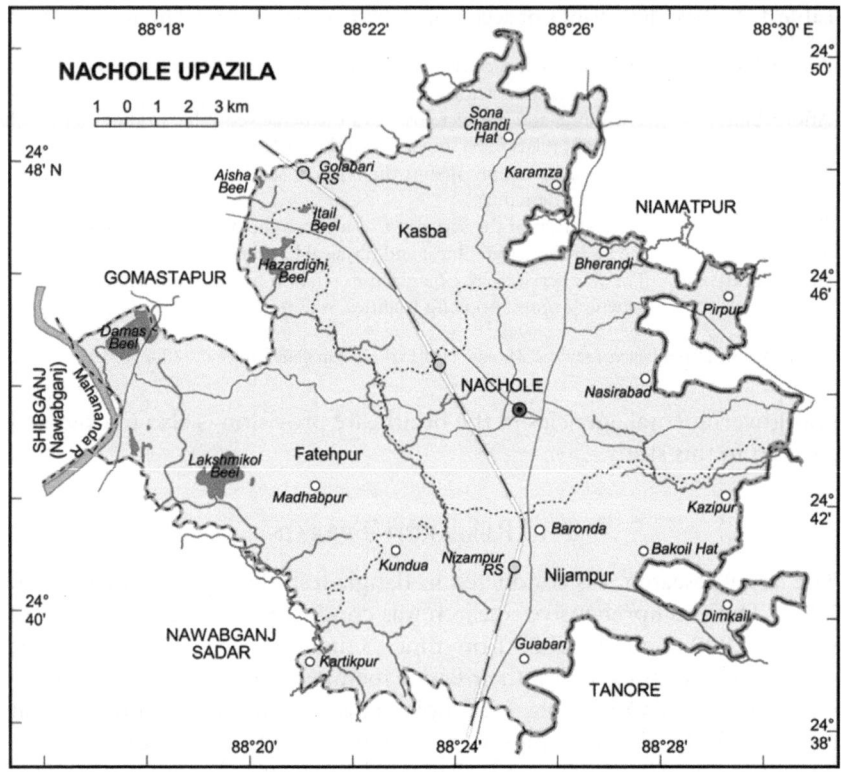

Fig. 1.1 Map of Nachol Upazila. (Source: Bangladesh National Portal, n.d.)

A sociological case-study design was chosen for this study. A sociological case study design is appropriate when the focus of a research design is on society, social institutions, and social relationships, and a study seeks to "*examine the structure, development, interaction, and collective behavior of organized groups of individuals*" (Hancock & Algozzine, 2006, p. 32). As this study aims at exploring the differences in experiences among different identity groups (gender and ethnicity) and between healthcare institutions and the society, sociological case study design is the proper design for this study among many other case study designs including ethnography, collective case study design, historical case study design, and exploratory case-study design.

The authors had no conflict of interest with the participants of the study. As researchers from Bangladesh, the authors have previous experience in conducting case-study research. Also, the researchers are familiar with the background, language, and culture of the study population. This helped the researchers throughout the study to address any unexpected occurrence. In this research, the structure of the local level healthcare delivery system, the interaction between the healthcare facilities and healthcare recipients, the collective health-seeking behavior of the Santal women, and the health crisis management during the COVID-19 outbreak have been studied (Fig. 1.2).

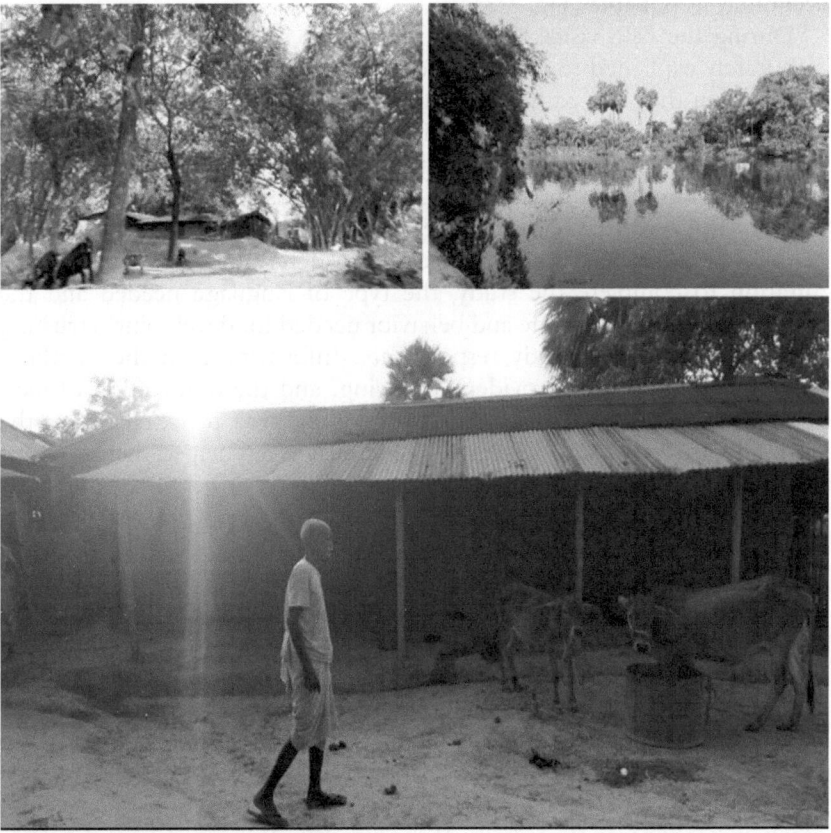

Fig. 1.2 Hakroil village in photos

The research had two sites in rural settings. One was in Hakroil village and the other in Paschim Lakkhanpur village of Nachol Upazila. The study areas were selected with great care so as to maximize the quality of the results. In order to select two villages for the present study, initially four villages were visited in the Nachol Upazila of Chapainawabganj district. Both villages correspond closely with the selection criteria set by the researchers. Both Hakroil and Paschim Lakkhanpur villages had an adequate number of ethnic women living. Moreover, the presence of NGOs who are running public healthcare programs was taken into consideration in the selection process. Both villages are more or less similar from all perspectives and this enabled the objectives of the research to be achieved as accurately as possible (Fig. 1.3).

During the field visits, the intention of the interviews was clearly and elaborately explained to the study respondents. They were aware that the information they shared would be used only for study purposes and they were free to participate or refrain from participating in this study. They were also informed that the information they shared would not impact or be used against them in any way. In the first instance of the research, a pilot study was carried out with a view to gain some general understanding of the field. The pilot study was helpful in determining a tentative time duration to complete the study, the type of language needed and the appropriate kind of attitude and behavior needed for developing a trusting relationship with the study respondents. Information on the unethical practices of the health providers, lobbying, and the domination of local power holders on the health service was very hard to extract from the respondents. However, this trusting relationship has helped them to overcome fear and share the information with the interviewer. The pilot study was also helpful in learning the attitude of the local people, rural cultural norms, and the local dialect.

The research conducted for this book has followed the triangulation method because a number of qualitative data collection techniques were used in this study, which has generated multiple perspectives from both ethnic women and the healthcare providers. Triangulation method ensures the validity of the empirical data and minimizes any potential biases of the researcher that may result from their prior knowledge, assumptions, or perceptions. The qualitative data collection tools used in this study include in-depth interviews, FGD and non-participant observations, application of which has ensured the validity of the research. Primary data of the study was collected from the Santal women, their family members (mostly

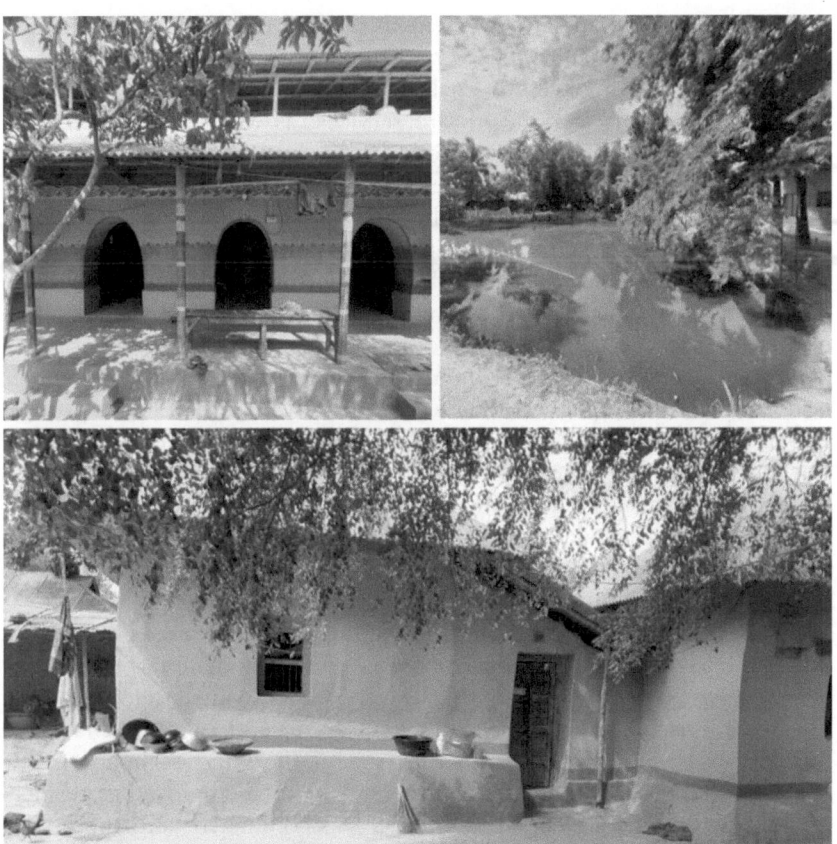

Fig. 1.3 Lakkhanpur village in photos

husbands), NGO officials, ethnic community leaders, local politicians, and non-ethnic women using in-depth interviews, focus group discussions, and non-participant observations. During interviews detailed case stories were also collected.

Santal women were chosen through purposive sampling for detailed interviewing. Purposive sample sizes are usually determined based on the theoretical saturation (Auerbach & Silverstein, 2003: 102). Theoretical saturation is a point in data collection when new data no longer adds new perceptions to the study. Santal women of this study were selected based on their availability and involvement in healthcare programs during the COVID-19 pandemic. Santal women were chosen for one-on-one in-depth interviews in order to analyze their experience of the available healthcare programs and healthcare services, as well as their ability to access healthcare. They were contacted directly. Only 40 ethnic women from the Santal tribe were interviewed because the saturation point was reached. Santal women were verbally invited to participate in an in-depth interview session. To support the analysis 40 Santal men (mostly the husbands and sons of the main respondents) and 40 non-ethnic women residing nearby were interviewed as well. The inclusion of Santal men and non-ethnic women has ensured a comprehensive analysis of the findings.

A total of 28 out of 40 women were interviewed separately in their house. The remaining 12 women were interviewed in three focus groups, two in their villages and one at the UHC. The UHC health providers were not allowed to be present during the interview session. Santal women were asked to answer a series of open-ended questions. The main aim of the in-depth interview was to collect qualitative data to examine the level of accessibility for ethnic women to healthcare. Each interview lasted approximately an hour.

The Focus Group Discussions (FGDs) for this study were conducted at Nachol Upazila Parishad, Hakroil village and Lakkhanpur village and involved participants who were exclusively Santal women, aged between 18 and 35 years. All of these participants were part of the Santal tribe residing in Nachol Upazila, and they shared the same occupation. For instance, FGD-1 was conducted with Santal women employed as cleaners at the Nachol Upazila Parishad, FGD-2 was conducted with those who worked as agriculture laborers and FGD-3 was conducted with homemakers. Each FGD session had a duration of 1.5–2 hours, allowing for in-depth discussions. To ensure that every participant had an opportunity to voice their thoughts and experiences, there were four participants in each FGD session.

During these FGD sessions, participants openly shared their collective experiences regarding healthcare access during the COVID-19 pandemic. They discussed how their socio-economic status was both influenced by and had an impact on the pandemic. Additionally, the discussions covered topics such as the types of discrimination they faced at public healthcare facilities, within their families, and in society at large. Furthermore, participants addressed the challenges they encountered as Santal women while seeking healthcare during the pandemic. They also shared insights on how they had successfully navigated and overcome these pandemic-related challenges. These FGDs served as a valuable platform for understanding the unique experiences and perspectives of these Santal women in the context of the COVID-19 pandemic.

In writing this book, Santal women and their narratives were mainly focused on. This book focuses on the healthcare access of rural ethnic women from the Santal tribe during the outbreak of COVID-19, the role of intersectional identity in influencing their healthcare accessibility, health-seeking behavior of rural Santal women during the COVID-19 pandemic and the limitations of the healthcare system of Bangladesh in ensuring equality in health service delivery. In writing this book, the authors did not insert their voice evidently in the text; rather, they tried to focus on the voice of Santal women and their stories.

OUTLINE OF THE BOOK

This chapter provides the foundation and background of the right to equal healthcare in Bangladesh. This chapter assesses the disproportionate healthcare effects of the pandemic on different vulnerable gender groups from an intersectional perspective in the global context. This chapter also examines the prevailing theoretical models on healthcare access in order to draw a theoretical foundation for the study. Adding to this, this chapter highlights various key concepts of the research that have been applied throughout the book, unveiling the conceptual perplexities. It also provides an overview of the research ground. It also discusses the research methods, research design, research sites, research processes, and ethical considerations. It provides the reasoning behind choosing the two selected villages.

Chapter 2 provides an overview of the healthcare system in Bangladesh. Focusing on the priorities of the healthcare policies of the Government of Bangladesh (GoB), this chapter explores the limitations of the existing healthcare policies. In addition, the roles of various health providers in Bangladesh have been examined to identify institutional limitations to ensure equal healthcare services for all.

Chapter 3 also highlights a range of literature relevant to the role of the healthcare services of Upazila Health Complexes (the first referral healthcare facilities at the local level) of Bangladesh and the healthcare accessibility of rural ethnic women, including the Santal women. The literature review identifies a gap in the current body of knowledge and methodological limitations of the previous research. Chapter 4 presents an overall analysis of Santal women's access to healthcare from an intersectional lens and the impact of COVID-19 on ethnic women's healthcare accessibility in rural Bangladesh. By exploring some of the issues experienced by the Santal women, a critical evaluation is made on their healthcare access during the pandemic in the light of a range of healthcare accessibility factors. To conduct an intersectional analysis, their experience and healthcare access is compared with that of ethnic men and non-ethnic women. In this chapter, the narratives of the respondents have been revealed that continue up to Chapter 5.

Chapter 5 highlights the challenges experienced by the Santal women in accessing healthcare during the pandemic as well as the institutional limitations in providing healthcare to all. This chapter analyzes how institutional, financial, and behavioral challenges limit Santal women's access to healthcare and limit their approachability to the healthcare facilities. This chapter describes how the health-seeking behavior of women and the behavior of the health providers shape the healthcare needs of Santal women. This chapter sheds light on socio-economic challenges, behavioral issues determining healthcare needs, and the institutional incapacity that have hindered the healthcare access of rural ethnic women during the pandemic.

Chapter 6 is the concluding chapter. This chapter summarizes the key findings of the study in the light of key research questions outlined in the first chapter. It also discusses how these findings fit into the current body of knowledge and highlights how they confirm, add to, and/or vindicate existing theories. This chapter also provides some policy recommendations based on the field investigation of the present study. And finally, it provides ideas about the scope of future research in fields relevant to this study.

References

Abdullah, D. (2022, February 1). Covid: Health rules openly disregarded at Sonamasjid land port. *Dhaka Tribune*. Retrieved September 25, 2023, from https://www.dhakatribune.com/bangladesh/health/286777/covid-health-rules-openly-disregarded-at

Akhtar, A. (2020, September 29). Filipinos make up 4% of nurses, but 31.5% of US COVID-19 nurse deaths. *The Business Insider*. https://www.businessinsider.com/filipinos-make-up-disproportionate-covid-19-nurse-deaths-2020-9

Al-Zaman, M. S. (2020). Healthcare crisis in Bangladesh during the COVID-19 pandemic. *The American Journal of Tropical Medicine and Hygiene, 103*(4), 1357–1359. https://doi.org/https://doi.org/10.4269/ajtmh.20-0826

Auerbach, F., & Silverstein, L. B. (2003). *Qualitative data: Introduction to coding and analysis.* New York University Press.

Aziz, A., Islam, M. M., & Zakaria, M. (2020). COVID-19 exposes digital divide, social stigma, and information crisis in Bangladesh. *Media Asia, 47*(3–4), 144–151.

Bangladesh National Portal. (n.d.). *Manchitre Nachol.* Bangladesh National Portal. Retrieved from https://shorturl.at/bl248

Behar, U. (2020). *Did COVID-19 widen the access gap for rural menstruators?* Retrieved July 4, 2023, from https://www.youthkiawaaz.com/2020/06/periods-do-not-stop-for-pandemics-2/

CDC. (2021). *10 essential public health services – CSTLTS.* Retrieved June 23, 2022, from https://www.cdc.gov/publichealthgateway/publichealthservices/essentialhealthservices.html

Chowdhury, S., Urme, S. A., Nyehn, B. A., Mark, H. R., Hassan, M. T., Rashid, S. F., Harris, N. B., & Dean, L. (2022). Pandemic portraits—An intersectional analysis of the experiences of people with disabilities and caregivers during COVID-19 in Bangladesh and Liberia. *Social Sciences, 11*(9), 378. https://doi.org/10.3390/socsci11090378

Darney, B. G., Aiken, A. R. A., & Küng, S. (2017). Access to contraception in the context of zika: Health system challenges and responses. *Obstetrics and Gynecology, 129*(4), 638–642.

Dhaka Tribune. (2020, March 23). Coronavirus: Bangladesh declares public holiday from March 26 to April 4. Retrieved September 25, 2023, from https://www.dhakatribune.com/bangladesh/204680/coronavirus-bangladesh-declares-public-holiday

Ellington, S., Strid, P., Tong, V. T., Woodworth, K., Galang, R. R., Zambrano, L. D., Nahabedian, J., Anderson, K., & Gilboa, S. M. (2020). *Morbidity and mortality weekly report characteristics of women of reproductive age with laboratory-confirmed SARS-CoV-2 infection by pregnancy status-United States.* Retrieved November 14, 2022, from https://www.cdc.gov/mmwr/mmwr_continuingEducation.html; https://www.cdc.gov/coronavirus/2019-ncov/cases-updates/cases-in-us.html

Foyez, A. (2021, August 2). Corruption in Bangladesh health sector on due to poor action. *The New Age BD.* Retrieved December 3, 2023, from https://www.newagebd.net/article/145287/corruption-in-bangladesh-health-sector-on-due-to-poor-action

George, I., & Kuruvilla, M. (2021). Introduction: Gender dimensions of COVID-19. In I. George & M. Kuruvilla (Eds.), *Gendered experiences of COVID-19 in India.* Palgrave Macmillan. https://doi.org/10.1007/978-3-030-85335-8_1

Gulliford, M., Figueroa-Munoz, J., Morgan, M., Hughes, D., Gibson, B., Beech, R., & Hudson, M. (2002). What does "access to health care" mean? *Journal of Health Services Research & Policy, 7*(3), 186–188.

Hancock, D. R., & Algozzine, R. (2006). *Doing case study research: A practical guide for beginning researchers.* Teachers College Press.

Hannon, E., Hanbali, L., Lehtimaki, S., & Schwalbe, N. (2022). Why we still need a pandemic treaty. *The Lancet Global Health, 10*(9).

Haque, N. T. (2021, May 26). What caused the Covid-19 surge in Chapainawabganj? *Dhaka Tribune.* Retrieved September 25, 2023, from https://www.dhaka-tribune.com/bangladesh/nation/247719/what-caused-the-covid-19-surge-in-chapainawabganj

Islam, M. R., & Hossain, M. J. (2021). Increments of gender-based violence amid COVID-19 in Bangladesh: A threat to global public health and women's health. *The International Journal of Health Planning and Management, 36*(6).

Islam, M. Z., Zaman, F., Farjana, S., & Khanam, S. (2019). Accessibility to health care services of Upazila Health Complex: Experience of rural people. *Journal of Preventive and Social Medicine, 38*(2), 30–37.

Kumar, B., & Pinky, S. D. (2021). Addressing economic and health challenges of COVID-19 in Bangladesh: Preparation and response. *Journal of Public Affairs, 21*(4).

Levesque, J. F., Harris, M. F., & Russell, G. (2013). Patient-centered access to health care: Conceptualizing access at the interface of health systems and populations. *International Journal for Equity in Health, 12*(1).

Malakoane, B., Heunis, J. C., Chikobvu, P., Kigozi, N. G., & Kruger, W. H. (2020). Public health system challenges in the Free State, South Africa: A situation appraisal to inform health system strengthening. *BMC Health Services Research, 20*(1), 1–14.

Mannan, M. A. (2013). Access to public health facilities in Bangladesh: A study on facility utilisation and burden of treatment. *The Bangladesh Development Studies, 36*(4).

Morgan, R., Pimenta, D. N., & Rashid, S. (2022). Gender equality and COVID-19: Act now before it is too late. *The Lancet, 399*(10344), 2327–2329.

Nicola, M., Alsafi, Z., Sohrabi, C., Kerwan, A., Al-Jabir, A., Iosifidis, C., Agha, M., & Agha, R. (2020). The socio-economic implications of the coronavirus pandemic (COVID-19): A review. *International Journal of Surgery, 78*, 185–193.

Pallegedara, A., & Grimm, M. (2017). Demand for private healthcare in a universal public healthcare system: Empirical evidence from Sri Lanka. *Health Policy and Planning, 32*(9), 1267–1284.

Penchansky, R., & Thomas, J. W. (1981). The Concept of Access. *Medical Care, 19*(2), 127–140. https://doi.org/10.1097/00005650-198102000-00001

Rasul, G., Nepal, A. K., Hussain, A., Maharjan, A., Joshi, S., Lama, A., Gurung, P., Ahmad, F., Mishra, A., & Sharma, E. (2021). Socio-economic implications of COVID-19 pandemic in South Asia: Emerging risks and growing challenges. *Frontiers in Sociology, 6.*

Rumi, M. H., Makhdum, N., Rashid, M. H., & Muyeed, A. (2021). Patients' satisfaction on the service quality of Upazila Health Complex in Bangladesh. *Journal of Patient Experience, 8.*

Ryan, N. E., & El Ayadi, A. M. (2020). A call for a gender-responsive, intersectional approach to address COVID-19. *Global Public Health, 15*(9), 1404–1412.

Schmitt, N. M., & Schmitt, J. (2008). Definition of public health. *Encyclopedia of Public Health, 1,* 222–233.

The Daily Star. (2021, June 13). 14-day lockdown: Covid-19 infection rate declining in Chapainawabganj. Retrieved September 25, 2023, from https://www.thedailystar.net/coronavirus-deadly-new-threat/news/14-day-lockdown-covid-19-infection-rate-declining-chapainawabganj-2110173

Ullah, A. A., & Chattoraj, D. (2022). *COVID-19 pandemic and the migrant population in Southeast Asia: Vaccine, diplomacy and disparity* (World Scientific Series on International Relations and Comparative Politics in Southeast Asia: Volume 2). https://doi.org/10.1142/12761

Ullah, A. A., Nawaz, F., & Chattoraj, D. (2021). Locked up under lockdown: The COVID-19 pandemic and the migrant population. *Social Sciences & Humanities Open, 3*(1), 100126. https://doi.org/10.1016/j.ssaho.2021.100126

UNHCHR. (2008, June). The Right to Health: Fact Sheet No. 31. Published by UNHCHR. Printed at United Nations, Geneva. ISSN 1014-5567. Retrieved from https://www.ohchr.org/sites/default/files/Documents/Publications/Factsheet31.pdf

WHO. (2019a). *Delivered by women, led by men: A gender and equity analysis of the global health and social workforce.* Retrieved October 21, 2022, from https://apps.who.int/iris/bitstream/handle/10665/311322/9789241515467-eng.pdf?sequence=1&isAllowed=y

WHO. (2019b). *Health emergency and disaster risk management framework.* Retrieved October 21, 2022, from https://apps.who.int/iris/bitstream/handle/10665/326106/9789241516181-eng.pdf?sequence=1&isAllowed=y

WHO. (2020). *The private health sector: An operational definition.* Retrieved November 15, 2022, from https://www.who.int/docs/default-source/health-system-governance/private-health-sector-an-operational-definition.pdf

CHAPTER 2

Equality and Inclusivity in the Healthcare System of Bangladesh

Abstract This chapter presents an overview discussion of the healthcare delivery system of Bangladesh, the institutional arrangements, the major gender-related health policies of the government, the key actors of healthcare delivery at the central to the local level, and the barriers to equal access to healthcare services in Bangladesh. The legal liability of healthcare provision, the institutional arrangements, the local level public healthcare service, the role of private and non-governmental actors in public healthcare provision, the government's attempts to promote inclusivity through healthcare policies, and finally the outcome and shortcomings of the present health policies of the Government of Bangladesh (GoB) are briefly discussed in this chapter. The weaknesses of current health policies and institutions to address the healthcare needs and challenges experienced by ethnic women are also highlighted.

Keywords Access • Equality • Institutional arrangements • Healthcare policy

This chapter begins by introducing the legal basis for equal healthcare in Bangladesh. It further explores the institutional arrangements of healthcare service delivery, and it then goes on to discuss the key actors and major limitations in the healthcare system of Bangladesh. This chapter reveals the legal obligations of the GoB to provide healthcare services to all its citizens and the limitations of the healthcare policies that restrict Santal women from accessing healthcare.

WHO HAS HEALTHCARE ACCESS IN BANGLADESH?

It is recognized in the constitution of the People's Republic of Bangladesh that healthcare is a fundamental requirement and the state is responsible for ensuring primary healthcare to its citizens. According to Article 15(a) of the constitution, the provision of medical care along with other basic necessities including food, clothing, shelter, and education is the responsibility of the State. Article 16 of the constitution has emphasized the development of public health in rural areas and removing disparity in the living standard between rural and urban areas. Article 18(1) specifies the provision of public healthcare as a primary role of the state. Along with these provisions, Article 28 of the Constitution of the GoB provides the foundation for equal rights to the citizens of the country regardless of religion, race, caste, sex, disability, or place of birth. Despite these constitutional principles, women experience inequality in their access to healthcare. The GoB has undertaken some additional policies and plans to address this gender gap in healthcare.

The National Health Policy of 2011 aims at ensuring accessibility of primary healthcare and emergency care for all citizens, ensuring quality healthcare services for all based on equity, and extending the coverage of quality healthcare services. In 2014, the Ministry of Health and Family Welfare (MoHFW) formulated a Gender Equity Strategy (GES)-2014. The mission of this strategy was to create and nurture a healthcare system that can provide equitable and quality healthcare (preventive, rehabilitative, and curative) for all citizens of the country. The strategy aimed to improve public health by ensuring better utilization of healthcare services, especially for women, children, adolescents, socially excluded and geographically marginalized populations, and poor people. In addition, MoHFW has formulated the National Population Policy, 2012; Healthcare Financing Strategy 2012–2032; National Nutrition Policy, 2015; National Drug Policy, 2016; Bangladesh National Strategy for Maternal Health 2015–2030; and National Strategy for Adolescent Health 2017.

A few other important policy documents provided important policy directions for public healthcare in Bangladesh. One notable mention is the "Eighth Five Year Plan (July 2020–June 2025): Promoting Prosperity and Fostering Inclusiveness" (hereinafter the 8th FYP) undertaken in a post-COVID-19 world, which expressed commitment to increase health-care funding and public–private cooperation in the healthcare sector. Strengthening the district-level healthcare facilities is another priority of this policy document. Healthcare schemes to fund Universal Health Care are planned to be introduced through this five-year plan. Increasing access for rural and urban populations to safe sanitation and drinking water is also prioritized. The social inclusion strategies of the 8th five-year plan are focused on the inclusion of children, disabled, Dalit and sex workers, and ethnic people living in the Chittagong Hill Tracts (CHT). Promoting inclusivity of ethnic communities of plain lands is absent from this policy document.

Despite these policy efforts by the GoB, Bangladesh has ranked the lowest in the first-ever Health Inclusivity Index 2022 by the Economist Impact (based in the United Kingdom), which measures the progress of inclusivity in healthcare in 40 countries. This report was prepared considering three key domains such as health in society, inclusive health systems, and people and community empowerment. This report reveals that most other countries in this study have laid emphasis on well-being, whereas Algeria, Bangladesh, Cuba, and Egypt ignored the notion of 'well-being' in their national health strategies (Uddin, 2022). Although inclusivity is not included in the national health strategy of Bangladesh, the GoB and NGOs have undertaken some measures in healthcare promotion that are likely to increase inclusivity in the health service delivery in the country, both by public and private actors. But the policy directives by the GoB remain ineffective in promoting inclusivity in healthcare accessibility.

These policy documents also reveal the weakness of the healthcare system and the inability of the public health system of Bangladesh to deal with complex viruses such as COVID-19. These inefficiencies and incapability together make the provision of inclusive healthcare challenging for the GoB. The GoB has undertaken a project called *Shastho Shurokkha Kormosuchi* to ensure universal health coverage in 2016. This project has been working tirelessly to improve the health status of women and girls. Through this project, healthcare infrastructure was developed and attempts were made to reach the marginalized population with healthcare services. Through this project, the GoB aims to achieve universal healthcare by the year 2032. This project is active in nine upazilas right now (Green Delta hosts, 2022).

THE STRUCTURE OF BANGLADESH'S HEALTHCARE
DELIVERY SYSTEM

The healthcare system of Bangladesh is a highly centralized, pluralistic system where four major actors drive and manage the structure and operations of the health sector. These actors include government, private sector, non-governmental organizations (NGOs), and donor agencies (Masud Ahmed et al., 2015). The whole healthcare system of Bangladesh is arranged under the leadership of the Ministry of Health and Family Welfare (MoHFW) with little authority delegated to its local-level counterparts. The MoHFW implements its policies and programs regarding healthcare provision with the aid of its executing and regulatory counterparts. The executing authorities under the MoHFW consist of five Directorates of the Ministry and some other organizations, namely— Health Services, Family Planning, Drug Administration, Nursing Services, and the Health Engineering Department. The regulatory authorities of the health sector are the Bangladesh Medical and Dental Council (BMDC), Bangladesh Nursing Council (BNC), State Medical Faculty (SMF), the Ayurvedic, Homeopathy, and Unani Board, and the Bangladesh Pharmacy Council (Masud Ahmed et al., 2015).

The MoHFW manages the healthcare system through the Directorate General of Health Services (DGHS) and the Directorate General of Family Planning (DGFP). These two Directorates General provide healthcare services to the people through district and general hospitals at the district level, Upazila Health Complexes at the sub-district level, Union Health and Family Welfare Centers at the union level, and community clinics at the village level. Along with the MoHFW-led system at the district, sub-district, and union levels, the Ministry of Local Government, Rural Development, and Cooperatives provides healthcare through urban primary care services. The local level parts of the organizational structure of the healthcare system of Bangladesh are—city corporations; local NGOs or private providers; Maternal and Child Welfare Centres (MCWC); Union Health and Family Welfare Centres (UHF & WC); district and general/specialized hospitals; Upazila Health Complex (UHC); union sub-centers (USC); rural sub-Centers (RSC); and community clinics (CC) (Sattar, 2021) (Figs. 2.1 and 2.2).

At the local level of the health system, primary care is provided through 432 UHCs, 3161 Union Health Centers, 1469 union sub-centers, 79 Union Health and Family Welfare Centers, and 14045 community clinics.

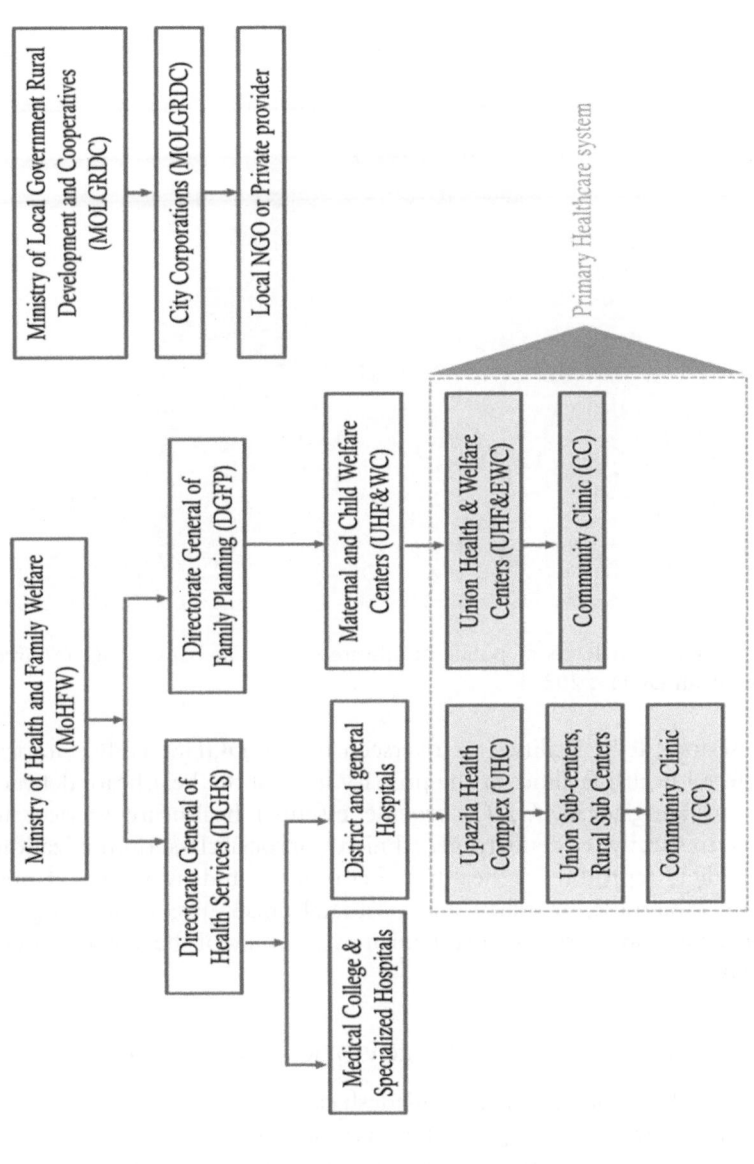

Fig. 2.1 The healthcare system of Bangladesh. (Source: Adapted from Masud Ahmed et al., 2015)

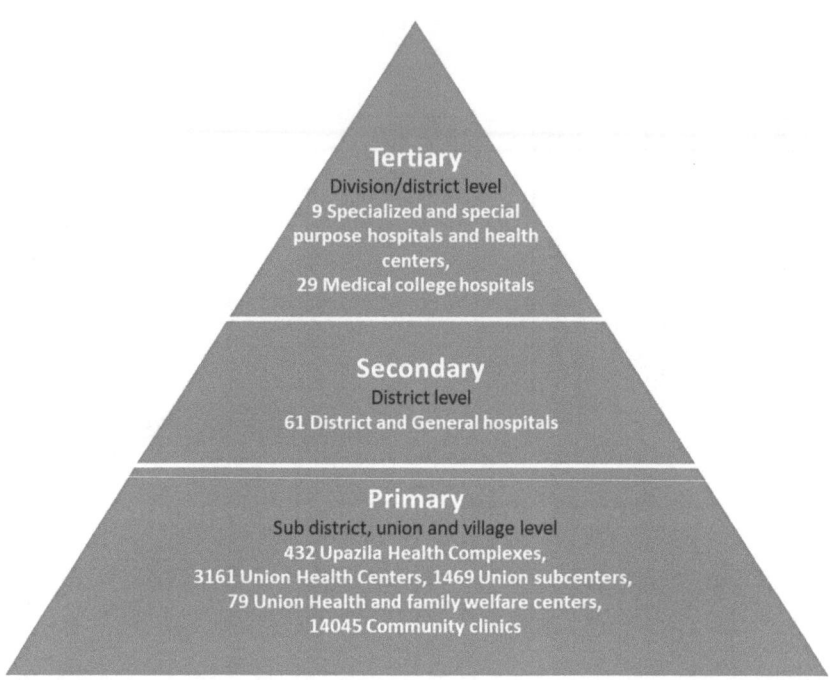

Fig. 2.2 Different levels of public healthcare services in Bangladesh. (Source: Adapted from DGHS, 2022)

All these local-level facilities are overseen by the DGHS. UHCs are the first referral health facilities at the primary level of the healthcare delivery system in Bangladesh. UHCs provide essential healthcare services to patients irrespective of gender, age, ethnicity, or social class. Immunization, healthy diet, reproductive healthcare education and awareness, family planning awareness, antenatal and postnatal check-ups, minor surgery, and the provision of free-of-cost medicines are some of the key services of the UHCs.

PRIVATE HEALTHCARE PROVIDERS IN BANGLADESH

Private healthcare providers in Bangladesh can be grouped into two broad categories. In the first category, there are organized for-profit and non-profit organizations with qualified health professionals. These private healthcare facilities include privately owned medical colleges, hospitals, clinics, diagnostic centers, laboratories, and drug stores. Private health service institutions are usually located in urban areas due to profit concerns. This often results in geographic inequity in health services (Sattar, 2021). The second category of the private healthcare system is the informal sector, which consists of untrained and unqualified healthcare providers. These alternative private providers include untrained allopaths, homeopaths, *kobiraj*, and village quacks (Sattar, 2021). Along with these private healthcare facilities, the NGOs, INGOs, and development partners of the GoB play a crucial role in both the public and private healthcare sectors of the country. NGOs and development partners participate in the health sector as direct providers and donors, as well as through healthcare awareness and advocacy programs.

Another key player in health provision in Bangladesh is the NGO sector. Bangladesh is well known for the wide range of NGOs working in the country. Although most of the NGOs are working to achieve financial solvency, empowerment, education, and climate issues, there are as many as 4000 NGOs that are working in the population, health, and nutrition sectors (Sattar, 2021). NGOs' operations in the health sector of Bangladesh are not limited to preventive and curative healthcare services. NGO services also cover healthcare advocacy, research, awareness building, nutrition, environmental health, and behavior change communication (Bhuiya, 2021). NGOs and development agencies in Bangladesh work in the areas of reproductive health, modern contraceptive use, antenatal care, skilled birth attendants, postnatal care, infant and breast-feeding practices, dissemination of knowledge and awareness of satellite and static clinics, and promoting optimal health behaviors (USAID, 2016).

Historically Christian missionary hospitals play a notable role in healthcare provision to the poor and marginalized community people of Bangladesh. Their operations among the ethnic and indigenous people of Bangladesh have been significant since the 1960s. Some of their noteworthy contributions lie in the area of maternal death reduction, providing primary healthcare service; low-cost, affordable, and quality health service provision; producing and training midwives; rural health workers; village doctors; and traditional birth attendants. The activities of the Christian missions have prioritized the healthcare needs of pregnant women, lactating mothers, and children (Shikdar, 2022). Over the years, the reputation of these Christian missionary hospitals has grown due to quality healthcare and the quality and behavior of the healthcare providers in these facilities (Rahman et al., 2012).

Along with the NGOs, many bilateral and multilateral development partners and donor agencies actively participate in the financing and planning of healthcare in the country. For instance, the World Bank and the Asian Development Bank (ADB) have signed agreements worth $100 million each for strengthening government systems for COVID-19 response (Hossain & Ahmed, 2020). The United States Agency for International Development (USAID) has donated a total of 18 freezer trucks to GoB, which are adequately equipped with cold-storage equipment in order to transport millions of COVID-19 vaccine doses across the country (US Embassy in Bangladesh, 2021). Sweden recently declared to provide $10 million to strengthen the quality of and access to midwives and comprehensive sexual and reproductive health services in Bangladesh, especially in the remote areas that are affected by climate change (Sweden to give, 2022).

Unraveling the Challenges of the Healthcare System in Bangladesh

The healthcare sector of Bangladesh is crippled by inadequate human resources and equipment, corruption, a low healthcare budget leading to high out-of-pocket payments, and a lack of cooperation among different public health authorities. Poor implementation of the health policies of the GoB at the local level adds weight to the problem. These institutional inefficiencies thrive as the prevailing social practice encourages the marginalization of poor, disadvantaged ethnic women from mainstream healthcare services. Because of these factors, the health policies of Bangladesh remain inefficient in addressing the healthcare needs of ethnic women and fail to promote inclusivity. Some of the key challenges facing the public healthcare system in Bangladesh are critically discussed in the following section.

The 8th FYP of Bangladesh has identified some of the major inequities in Bangladesh's health and nutrition services. These challenges include high mortality rates due to non-communicable diseases (NCDs); high out-of-pocket expenditure; poor coverage and low quality of essential nutrition services; inadequate facility readiness, including the Electronic Logistic Management Information System (E-LMIS); inefficient service quality and coverage; poor regulation and management of the private sector; stagnant healthcare allocation; the absence of a health insurance system in the public healthcare system; and poor quality of healthcare. A number of studies on the healthcare system of Bangladesh have revealed similar challenges as barriers to access to healthcare services and inclusivity for ethnic and backward people to public healthcare services.

Molla and Chi (2017), for instance, have reported that health system financing in Bangladesh is characterized by high out-of-pocket (OOP) payments (63.3% and increasing) and thus impacts different social classes unequally. High OOP payments result in partial care aggravating the disease condition, selling assets to manage the treatment costs, becoming malnourished by decreasing food consumption, and so on (Molla & Chi, 2017). Along with high OOP healthcare payments, health insurance in Bangladesh remains virtually non-existent (Khan, 2022). Together, these two phenomena create an environment where equitable access to healthcare only exists in texts; but in reality, people with greater resources enjoy better healthcare services, while those with stagnant family incomes end up in greater poverty. This condition got worse during the COVID-19 outbreak as the compulsory lockdown measures, while essential to prevent the spread of the virus, have had unequal impacts, leaving some in significantly worse situations than others (Hebbar et al., 2020).

Poor cooperation between different government agencies regarding public health service delivery is another key challenge to the health system of Bangladesh. There are ambiguities between the Ministry of Health and Family Welfare (MoHFW) and the Ministry of Local Government, Rural Development, and Co-operatives (MoLGRDC) regarding the roles and responsibilities of urban health (Sattar, 2021). While the MoHFW is responsible for overseeing the overall health system of Bangladesh, the MoLGRDC is responsible for looking after urban and public health issues. Activities of MoLGRDC relating to public health involve expanding access to urban primary healthcare services, strengthening municipal public health governance, enhancing food and water safety, and improving urban waste management. Ambiguities arise when the functions of these two ministries overlap, especially in the areas of safe water and sanitation, medical services, promotion of public health awareness and health education, hospital and dispensary management, vaccination and community health, and prevention of infectious and communicable diseases.

Apart from the above mentioned, corruption, mismanagement of resources, irregularities in institutional capacities, and finally poor healthcare governance remain key barriers to healthcare accessibility for the disadvantaged poor people of Bangladesh. While the quality of the health services provided by public healthcare facilities remains poor and inaccessible, private sector facilities are often unregulated (Sattar, 2021). In 2022 alone, the GoB will have shut down more than 1600 illegal healthcare institutions. But there is no accurate estimation of the actual number of unregistered hospitals, clinics, diagnostic centers, and blood banks that exist in the country (Hasan, 2022). Along with this, even though the number of physicians in Bangladesh is on the rise, there is still a significant gap in the doctor-to-patient ratio. As of 2019, there was only one doctor for about 1667 people in Bangladesh (World Bank, 2019). Thus, Bangladesh struggles to ensure healthcare for all as the number of healthcare providers is way behind demand.

REFERENCES

Bhuiya, S. (2021, January 8). NGOs in the health sector of Bangladesh. *The Daily Asian Age.* https://dailyasianage.com/news/251820/ngos-in-health-sector-of-bangladesh

DGHS. (2022). *Organization registry.* Retrieved October 16, 2022, from http://facilityregistry.dghs.gov.bd/report_org_list.phpp

Green Delta hosts a universal health coverage seminar. (2022, November 23). *The Business Standard.* https://www.tbsnews.net/economy/corporates/g100-green-delta-hosts-universal-health-coverage-seminar-5374466

Hasan, R. A. (2022, December 12). Who benefits from the raids at healthcare facilities? *The Daily Star.* https://www.thedailystar.net/opinion/views/news/who-Benefits-the-raids-healthcare-facilities-3141081

Hebbar, P. B., Sudha, A., Dsouza, V., Chilgod, L., & Amin, A. (2020). Healthcare delivery in India amid the Covid-19 pandemic: Challenges and opportunities. *Indian Journal of Medical Ethics,* 1–4. https://doi.org/10.20529/IJME.2020.064

Hossain, M. R., & Ahmed, S. (2020). A case for building a stronger health care system in Bangladesh. Retrieved December 6, 2022, from https://blogs.worldbank.org/endpovertyinsouthasia/case-building-stronger-health-care-system-bangladesh

Khan, M. T. H. (2022, November 13). Envisioning universal health coverage in Bangladesh. *The Daily Star.* https://www.thedailystar.net/star-health/news/envisioning-Universal-health-coverage-bangladesh-31677666

Masud Ahmed, S., Alam, B. B., Anwar, I., Begum, T., Huque, R., Khan, J. A. M., Nababan, H., Osman, F. A., Naheed, A., & Hort, K. (2015). Bangladesh health system review. *Health Systems in Transition, 5*(3).

Molla, A. A., & Chi, C. (2017). Who pays for healthcare in Bangladesh? An analysis of progressivity in health systems financing. *International Journal for Equity in Health, 16*(1), 1–10.

Rahman, S. A., Tara Kielmann, B. M. P., & Normand, C. (2012). Healthcare-seeking behavior among the tribal people of Bangladesh: Can the current health system really meet their needs? *Journal of Health, Population, and Nutrition, 30*(3), 353.

Sattar, M. P. (2021). Health sector governance: An overview of the legal and institutional framework in Bangladesh. *Open Journal of Social Sciences, 9*(11), 395–414.

Shikdar, S. (2022, May 20). Healthcare delivery in a remote corner. *The Financial Express.* https://thefinancialexpress.com.bd/views/healthcare-delivery-in-a-remote-corner-16530691255

Sweden to give $10 million to UNFPA to support midwifery, reproductive health in Bangladesh. (2022, October 24). *The Daily Star.* https://www.thedailystar.net/health/news/sweden-give-10-million-unfpa-support-Midwifery-reproductive-health-bangladesh-31507666

The World Bank. (2019). *Physicians (per 1,000 people)—Bangladesh.* Retrieved December 20, 2022, from https://data.worldbank.org/indicator/SH.MED.PHYS.ZS?locations=BD

Uddin, S. (2022, October 13). BD scores lowest among 40 nations. *The Financial Express.* https://thefinancialexpress.com.bd/health/bd-scores-lowest-among-40-nations-1665625619

US Embassy in Bangladesh. (2021). *United States donates 18 freezer trucks for COVID-19 vaccine delivery in Bangladesh—U.S. Embassy in Bangladesh.* Retrieved December 3, 2022, from https://bd.usembassy.gov/united-states-donates-18-freezer-trucks-for-covid-19-vaccine-delivery-in-bangladesh/

USAID. (2016). *Bangladesh nongovernmental organization health service delivery project—2014 baseline rural survey.* Retrieved December 6, 2022, from https://www.measureevaluation.org/resources/publications/tr-16-125a/at_download/document

CHAPTER 3

Healthcare Access and Ethnic Women's Right to Health: A Void in the Literature

Abstract This chapter elucidates a range of theoretical frameworks concerning healthcare accessibility and serves as a foundational underpinning for the present study. As the healthcare delivery system has grown more intricate and inclusivity has gained prominence within global healthcare policies, the models addressing healthcare accessibility have evolved into a more intricate construct. However, a substantial number of these accessibility models have overlooked the multifaceted identity factors inherent to individuals seeking services, thereby neglecting a comprehensive analysis of healthcare access. Within this context, the chapter accentuates the constraints inherent in prevailing healthcare accessibility models. It underscores noteworthy arguments and constraints within the body of literature concerning ethnic women's access to healthcare services at the local level in Bangladesh. Through a comprehensive literature review, this study identifies a discernible gap in the present comprehension of this issue. Furthermore, the review critically assesses both the methodological and conceptual limitations underpinning existing research endeavors in this domain.

Keywords Theoretical framework • Access to healthcare • Public health • Public healthcare

F. Nawaz, AN Bushra, *Santal Women and the Health Care Regime*, https://doi.org/10.1007/978-3-031-48872-6_3

This chapter serves as the foundational underpinning of the present book. Within this chapter, various models pertaining to healthcare accessibility are examined, revealing their limitations in effectively addressing healthcare access and requirements of ethnic women. It illuminates how the intersection of their ethnic and gender identities significantly influences their access to healthcare. Surprisingly, the literature that has ventured into an analysis of the healthcare necessities and access of Santal women in Bangladesh through a theoretical framework is scarce. In response to this critical theoretical void, this chapter endeavors to amalgamate the intersectionality model with the healthcare access paradigm as it pertains to Santal women in Bangladesh. Furthermore, the evolving landscape of the COVID-19 pandemic has introduced an array of new and distinctive challenges, thereby establishing an entirely novel context within which healthcare accessibility can be studied. In light of this comprehensive theoretical foundation, this book emerges as a substantial contribution to the exploration of ethnic women and their healthcare accessibility amidst a global pandemic.

THEORETICAL MODELS ON ACCESS TO HEALTHCARE: A CRITICAL ANALYSIS

Theoretical discussion on people's accessibility to essential public services, including health services, has been a matter of concern in social justice, equitable public service delivery, and gender equity scholarships. Access to services, as explained by some scholars, is subject to several factors, such as demand and supply factors, tangible and intangible factors, location factors, social factors, and gender factors. At the same time, some scholars have seen access to healthcare from a behavioral perspective, while others have emphasized equitable healthcare, seeing it through the lens of social justice. For the purpose of this study, three popular theoretical models have been taken into critical consideration. These three models represent three dominant schools of thought in the existing studies on accessibility. Among these three models, Anderson's healthcare utilization model views access from the behavioral perspective of the service recipient, Crenshaw's intersectionality proposes a framework of socio-political and identity factors that shape people's experiences of inequality in the social and political realm; and finally, Levesque's conceptual framework of access to health conceptualizes access to healthcare from a demand-supply outlook where both socio-cultural and organizational determinants of access are taken into account.

Levesque's Conceptual Framework of Access to Health

Levesque et al. (2013) have conceptualized access by exploring five dimensions of it, capturing supply side and demand side determinants: (1) Approachability; (2) Acceptability; (3) Availability and Accommodation; (4) Affordability; and (5) Appropriateness. These five dimensions of accessibility are closely related to the five dimensions of ability of the service recipients, which include: (1) ability to perceive, (2) ability to seek, (3) ability to reach, (4) ability to pay, and (5) ability to engage. These determinants are influenced by ecological, financial, and organizational obstacles (Levesque et al., 2013) (Fig. 3.1).

This model, although able to explain the abuse and neglect initiated to discourage ethnic minorities from seeking healthcare, has certain limitations that make it unsuitable for the current study. As it lacks a feedback loop, this model fails to connect health outcomes with the healthcare needs and perceptions of the population. It also doesn't give any clear idea about the role of genetic, ethnic, and political factors in determining and influencing healthcare needs. Personal and social values, culture, gender,

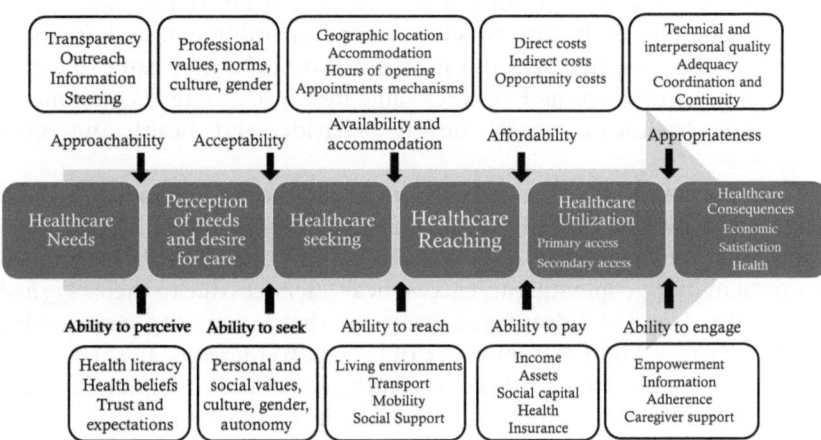

Fig. 3.1 Levesque's conceptual framework of access to health. (Source: Levesque et al., 2013)

and autonomy are taken into consideration as factors influencing people's ability to seek healthcare. But social identity (marginalized status) and health-seeking behavior are shaped by political realities as well as by existing power relations in a community, especially in developing countries where service delivery at the local level is subject to domination by the local political and power elites.

Ronald Andersen's Healthcare Utilization Model

Ronald M. Andersen's model of healthcare utilization is a behavioral model of access to healthcare that was first proposed in the 1970s and later developed in four phases to come into being in its present format in the 1990s. This model assumes that people's healthcare needs and perceptions of need are determined by predisposing characteristics (demographic, social structure, and health beliefs) and enabling resources (potential access: personal/family and community). After the need realization (perceived need and evaluated needs), the health behavior is dependent upon the personal health practice of the individual and the use of health services (realized access). Access to healthcare, here, can take either of two forms: (1) equitable access (determined by demographic characteristics and need) and (2) inequitable access (determined by social structure, health beliefs, and enabling resources). Health outcomes in this model are seen through the lenses of perceived health status, evaluated health status, and patient satisfaction. The healthcare system, external environment, and feedback loop are recent inclusions in this model that describe how external forces like politics, socio-cultural realities, and healthcare system components determine healthcare needs, health behavior, and health outcomes (Fig. 3.2).

This model, however, is appropriate in instances where adequate and functioning healthcare facilities are available for the community. There are cases where people's need for healthcare is realized and healthcare services are present, but people still can't access health services due to their assigned marginalized and disadvantaged status in the community, unfavorable location factors, and the dominance of local power groups. In such a situation, external factors directly constrain the use of health services, bypassing the need for them. Anderson's model fails to address this issue.

The existence of proper health policies and healthcare facilities alone is not enough for the effective implementation of equitable healthcare programs. The behavior of healthcare providers plays a big role in shaping

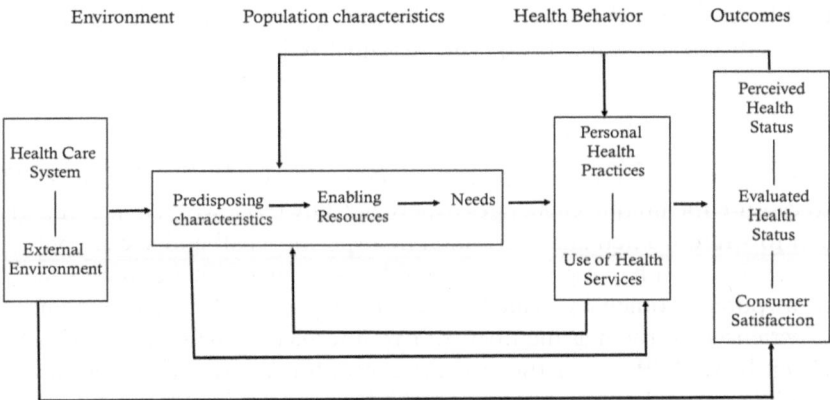

Fig. 3.2 Andersen's healthcare utilization model. (Source: Andersen, 1995, p. 8)

people's healthcare needs and perceived health status. Andersen emphasized the behavior of the service recipients in determining their access to health services but ignored the attitudes and behaviors of the healthcare providers. Empirical data suggest that inappropriate behavior and the poor image of health providers, especially among the disadvantaged, are key barriers for people to access healthcare even when the need is felt (Islam et al., 2019; Mohiuddin, 2020; Rumi et al., 2021).

Although the existing models of healthcare access provide a valuable framework for understanding accessibility issues, they have not fully accounted for an essential determinant that significantly influences people's perceptions and social experiences: the identity factor. Empirical studies focusing on gender, location, and economic disadvantage have been conducted to analyze healthcare access, but they often fall short in providing a comprehensive understanding of inequality. Inequality is frequently a result of multiple intersecting identity factors, necessitating an intersectional lens to fully comprehend it. Therefore, the two prevailing models of healthcare accessibility, while widely accepted, may not be entirely suitable for this study, which aims to offer a comprehensive view of healthcare access for economically disadvantaged ethnic women who experience overlapping forms of disadvantage. To address this issue adequately, this study adopts Crenshaw's intersectionality framework as its theoretical foundation. By incorporating intersectionality in the study of healthcare access, the study aims to better capture the complex dynamics of healthcare access for this specific marginalized group.

Kimberlé Crenshaw's Intersectionality

The term intersectionality was first coined by Kimberlé Crenshaw in 1989 to capture the unique challenges experienced by black women in comparison to white women and black men in a specific legal[1] and social context where the court had repeatedly treated black women either as purely black or as purely women but failed to see the expanded degree of inequities experienced by them as members of two intersecting marginalized groups (Crenshaw, 1989). Over the years, the term 'intersectionality' has gained much attention in discussions of racial injustice, identity politics, and policies. Crenshaw used intersectionality to denote how race, class, gender, and other systems of social identity combine to produce inequality by making room for privilege and discrimination (Crenshaw, 1991). Intersectionality challenges the notion that gender alone is the determining factor in the inequality experienced by women in the social and political spheres.

The underlying assumption of the intersectionality framework is that human beings are exposed to multiple identity factors that intersect and/ or overlap to produce a more complex identity, based on which they are either discriminated against or privileged in a socio-political setting. Intersectionality views a number of identities in combination rather than seeing each in isolation. Although the term has begun its journey to address sexual and racial injustice, it now encompasses other identity factors, including gender, sexuality, class, ability, nationality, citizenship, religion, and body type. In short, intersectionality is a prism to observe how multiple forms of inequality operate together and exacerbate one another (UN Women, 2020) (Fig. 3.3).

Evidence of previous pandemics shows that a pandemic affects individuals and social groups in a different manner based on contextual factors of marginalization, including gender, race or ethnicity, age, indignity,

---

[1] Crenshaw, in her paper "Demarginalizing the Intersection of Race and Sex", focused on three legal cases that dealt with the issues of both racial discrimination and sex discrimination, namely, *DeGraffenreid v. General Motors*, *Moore v. Hughes Helicopter, Inc.*, and *Payne v. Travenol*. In each case, Crenshaw argued that the legal system had forgotten that black women are both black and women and thus are discriminated against both their racial and their gender identities and often a combination of both.

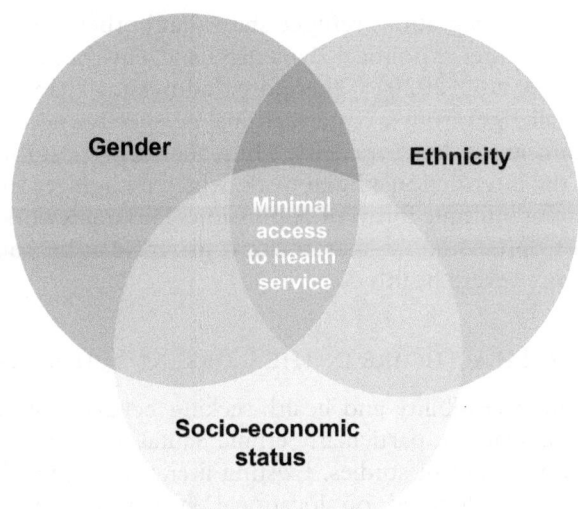

Fig. 3.3 Intersectional framework to study access to healthcare. (Source: Authors)

class, socio-economic status, geography, disability, sexuality, religion, migration/refugee status, and other structural conditions, including employment, and political and environmental stressors (Ryan & El Ayadi, 2020). In this regard, it is critical to address within-group heterogeneity in addressing pandemic-related healthcare challenges. Intersectionality, in the context of healthcare provision, is a useful tool to reveal intersectional factors that hinder the access of women belonging to more than one disadvantaged group. Thus, intersectionality is the best instrument to explore the key objectives of this study.

Andersen's Healthcare Utilization Model and Levesque's Conceptual Framework of Access to Health exhibit limitations in their capacity to promote inclusive healthcare access for individuals facing multiple disadvantages. Additionally, these models overlook the influence of various identity factors on healthcare outcomes for ethnic women in developing countries like Bangladesh. Previous pandemics have shown that pandemics affect individuals and social groups differently as they are influenced by contextual factors of marginalization such as gender, 'race'/ethnicity, age, indignity, class, socio-economic status, geography, disability, sexuality, religion, migration/refugee status, and other structural conditions like employment, political dynamics, and environmental stressors (Ryan & El Ayadi, 2020). Therefore, addressing pandemic-related healthcare challenges from an intersectional perspective necessitates considering within-group heterogeneity. Thus, the theoretical foundation of this study is the intersectional framework, which recognizes the interconnected nature of multiple forms of oppression. This framework posits that the effects of oppression on marginalized groups can be compounded, leading to more severe health disparities.

ETHNIC HEALTHCARE IN THE CURRENT SCHOLARSHIPS

The healthcare accessibility and health-seeking behavior of ethnic communities in Bangladesh, particularly ethnic Santal women, have received scant attention in current studies. Existing literature on equal healthcare has predominantly focused on locational factors, age groups, socioeconomic background, and gender, with transgender healthcare being almost absent from the research. While some studies have explored the healthcare access and needs of minority and disadvantaged groups, they often fail to adequately capture patient satisfaction with health services and identify institutional challenges in healthcare provision (Rumi et al., 2021; Mannan, 2013; Islam et al., 2019; Mohiuddin, 2020). Additionally, very few studies have included rural ethnic populations in discussions of overall healthcare services in rural Bangladesh. Moreover, existing literature on healthcare among different ethnic communities in Bangladesh primarily concentrates on those living in the Chittagong Hill Tracts (CHT), with limited attention to Santal communities residing in Northern Bangladesh, rendering them nearly absent from public health research (Tabassum, 2017; Rahman et al., 2012; Kabir et al., 2019; Rahman et al., 2021).

Tabassum's (2017) study on the role of mass media campaigns on the health behaviors of indigenous people in Bangladesh has delved into the health behaviors of indigenous communities and examined the impact of mass media on change in their health behaviors. The study's findings indicate that indigenous communities with limited health literacy exhibit reduced responsiveness to health-related information and an increased tendency to adopt unfavorable health behaviors such as tobacco usage, unhealthy dietary patterns, physical inactivity, and alcohol consumption.

The research identifies three primary challenges in redirecting the health behaviors of indigenous communities toward the prevention of Non-Communicable Diseases (NCDs) in Bangladesh. These challenges encompass a lack of awareness regarding the severity of these diseases, insufficient health literacy, and the absence of advocacy for health intervention programs targeting indigenous individuals affected by NCDs. This study identifies some challenges to the accessibility of healthcare for ethnic people in Bangladesh; however, it does not highlight the healthcare needs of ethnic women, and ethnic and gender identity were not the central concerns of this study.

Islam and Odland (2011) have examined the utilization of antenatal and postnatal care among Mru women through a mixed-methods study involving 374 married Mru women with young children from Bandarban District, Bangladesh. They found that traditional Mru prenatal and postnatal practices hindered the use of formal healthcare services. Antenatal and postnatal care visits were lower than the national average, with rural traditional midwives being the primary caregivers. Challenges in accessing care included travel distance and transportation issues. Multivariate analysis identified factors like residence, age, education, distance to service centers, and media exposure as influencing care-seeking behavior. The study highlights the role of cultural norms, geography, infrastructure, and socioeconomic status in shaping maternal healthcare behavior. Improving healthcare delivery and local-level education is crucial for enhancing maternal and child health in the Mru community.

Another study by Akter et al. (2020) looked into the barriers to accessing maternal healthcare (MHC) services by indigenous women in Bangladesh. The majority of the participants of this study were categorized as 'Users' as they accessed MHC services during their last pregnancy or childbirth. The remaining seven were categorized as 'Non-users' as they didn't use antenatal, facility delivery, or postnatal care. Participants expressed a preference for culturally relevant, respectful, home-based, and affordable care. Formal MHC services were often perceived as reserved for complications and emergencies. Barriers to accessing MHC services included low awareness, concerns about costs, limited transportation, and fear of intrusive practices. Negative experiences within health facilities, such as demands for unofficial payments and abusive treatment, discouraged women from seeking future MHC services. This study recommends that a comprehensive approach is needed that considers cultural values, priorities, and concerns in order to enhance MHC service access for indigenous women. Reforms in the area of healthcare access should address education, service delivery options, and community engagement to ensure culturally appropriate and flexible maternal healthcare.

In their study, Ali et al. (2016) explored the perceptions, diagnosis, and causes attributed to black fever, a tropical disease among Santal people. Indigenous communities hold diverse views on black fever, associating it with concepts such as a divine curse, dark forces, and black magic. Around 70% of Santal patients become aware of black fever through NGOs or medical tests. Among the Santal indigenous group, distinct physical characteristics linked to black fever are noted, including anger, chills, rice avoidance, headaches, anemia, stillbirths, abdominal enlargement, menstrual cessation, weight loss, and reduced strength. Knowledge about black fever varies, leading to delayed recognition. A belief in supernatural influences, the idea that it can be transmitted through touch, and concerns about social stigma affecting treatment are prevalent. About 78% of patients feel their limited understanding of black fever impacts the treatment process. After seeking treatment from NGOs or medical facilities, 45% of individuals reported no side effects, while the remaining experienced various side effects.

Underlying Research Gaps

Research on healthcare for ethnic communities in Bangladesh has highlighted several key challenges that limit their access to effective health services. One significant finding indicates that indigenous groups with low health literacy tend to be less receptive to health information, leading to the adoption of negative health behaviors, such as tobacco use, unhealthy diets, physical inactivity, and alcohol consumption. Additionally, three major obstacles have been identified in the healthcare access of indigenous communities: a lack of awareness regarding disease severity, insufficient health literacy, and a lack of advocacy for health intervention programs for those suffering from non-communicable diseases (Tabassum, 2017). Furthermore, culture and beliefs play a crucial role in determining healthcare service preferences for ethnic individuals. Many prefer informal sector providers like para-professionals and traditional healers due to their physical and cultural accessibility, particularly when public healthcare facilities are underutilized. The choice of therapy is influenced by individuals' perceptions of illness causes and their financial and physical ability to access health services (Uddin et al., 2013; Nawaz & Bushra, 2023).

In the context of mental healthcare, ethnic communities face difficulties accessing services for various reasons. Some individuals do not fully comprehend the importance of mental healthcare, while others worry about the expenses associated with such services and face transportation limitations. Moreover, a fear of intrusive procedures acts as a barrier to seeking mental healthcare. Additionally, some ethnic women have been discouraged from seeking healthcare due to unofficial payments demanded and mistreatment by public facility staff during previous health service experiences (Akter et al., 2020). Other studies have found that gender inequality and power dynamics at the community level significantly impact ethnic women's autonomy over their reproductive health. Cultural norms often compel women to submit to the decisions of their in-laws, working-age males, and elder women during the process of giving birth, and health-seeking (Tarafder & Sultan, 2014; Rahman et al., 2012; Kabir et al., 2019).

The existing literature on ethnic healthcare reveals inadequacies, primarily due to its predominantly quantitative nature, which hinders an in-depth analysis of healthcare access issues. While quantitative studies identify unequal access and varying impacts of healthcare emergencies on different gendered and ethnic groups, they lack substantial explanations for this disparity and overlook societal factors that contribute to it. Another drawback is the failure to effectively address within-group differences. Qualitative researches, often relying on secondary data rather than first-hand field experience, also exhibit limitations in providing comprehensive insights into complex gendered differentiation in healthcare accessibility. In contrast, the present empirical study adopts a qualitative approach, a novel addition to the methodology.

Remarkably, previous research has not employed an intersectional perspective to investigate health-seeking behavior, access to public healthcare services for ethnic women during COVID-19, the influence of power dynamics in health policy implementation, or the multi-dimensional experiences of inequality among impoverished ethnic women. By addressing these gaps, the current study enriches the existing knowledge base in this pertinent domain. Incorporating the COVID-19 pandemic context into the analysis of Upazila Health Complex (UHC) services is lacking in some studies. However, this research delves into the pandemic's impact on healthcare accessibility for Santal women, shedding light on how a public health emergency affects minority women and the challenges it presents in healthcare access. This valuable contribution to academic scholarship empowers researchers and policy analysts to develop improved healthcare crisis management strategies that are better equipped to address future uncertainties that may hinder healthcare access for marginalized communities and those residing in remote areas.

REFERENCES

Akter, S., Davies, K., Rich, J. L., & Inder, K. J. (2020). Barriers to accessing maternal health care services in the Chittagong Hill Tracts (CHT), Bangladesh: A qualitative descriptive study of Indigenous women's experiences. *PLoS One*, *15*(8). https://doi.org/10.1371/journal.pone.0237002

Ali, M. Y., Rahman, M. R., Javed, A., Toppo, A., & Akhtar, M. R. (2016). Indigenous santal people sense and etiology regarding black fever illness. *American Journal of Health Research*, *4*(5), 143.

Andersen, R. M. (1995). Revisiting the behavioral model and access to medical care: Does it matter? *Journal of Health and Social Behavior*, *36*(1), 1–10. https://doi.org/10.2307/2137284

Crenshaw, K. (1989). Demarginalizing the intersection of race and sex: A Black feminist critique of antidiscrimination doctrine, feminist theory and antiracist politics. *University of Chicago Legal Forum*, *1989*(1), 139–167.

Crenshaw, K. (1991). Mapping the margins: Intersectionality, identity politics, and violence against women of color. *Stanford Law Review*, *43*(6).

Islam, M. R., & Odland, J. O. (2011). Determinants of antenatal and postnatal care visits among Indigenous people in Bangladesh: A study of the Mru community. *Rural and Remote Health*, *11*(2).

Islam, M. Z., Zaman, F., Farjana, S., & Khanam, S. (2019). Accessibility to health care services of Upazila Health Complex: Experience of rural people. *Journal of Preventive and Social Medicine*, *38*(2), 30–37.

Kabir, A., Datta, R., Raza, S. H., & Louise Maitrot, M. R. (2019). Health shocks, care-seeking behavior and coping strategies of extreme poor households in Bangladesh's Chittagong Hill tracts (CHT). *BMC Public Health*, *19*(1008). https://doi.org/10.1186/s12889-019-7335-7

Levesque, J. F., Harris, M. F., & Russell, G. (2013). Patient-centered access to health care: Conceptualizing access at the interface of health systems and populations. *International Journal for Equity in Health*, *12*(1).

Mannan, M. A. (2013). Access to public health facilities in Bangladesh: A study on facility utilisation and burden of treatment. *The Bangladesh Development Studies*, *36*(4).

Mohiuddin, A. K. (2020). Patient satisfaction with healthcare services: Bangladesh perspective. *International Journal of Public Health Science*, *9*(1), 34–45.

Nawaz, F., & Bushra, A. N. (2023). Health-seeking behavior of rural ethnic women in Bangladesh: A critical analysis through an intersectional lens. *Arab Economic and Business Journal, 15*(2), 10.38039/2214-4625.1029.

Rahman, F. N., Khan, H. T. A., Hossain, M. J., & Iwuagwu, A. O. (2021). Health and wellbeing of indigenous older adults living in the tea gardens of Bangladesh. *PLoS One, 16*(3). https://doi.org/10.1371/journal.pone.0247957

Rahman, S. A., Tara Kielmann, B. M. P., & Normand, C. (2012). Healthcare-seeking behavior among the tribal people of Bangladesh: Can the current health system really meet their needs? *Journal of Health, Population and Nutrition, 30*(3), 353.

Rumi, M. H., Makhdum, N., Rashid, M. H., & Muyeed, A. (2021). Patients' satisfaction on the service quality of Upazila Health Complex in Bangladesh. *Journal of Patient Experience, 8*.

Ryan, N. E., & El Ayadi, A. M. (2020). A call for a gender-responsive, intersectional approach to address COVID-19. *Global Public Health, 15*(9), 1404–1412.

Tabassum, R. (2017). Health paradox of indigenous people in Bangladesh: Unraveling aspects of mass media campaigns in changing health behaviors to prevent non-communicable diseases. *South East Asia Journal of Public Health, 6*(2), 17–22.

Tarafder, T., & Sultan, P. (2014). Reproductive health beliefs and their consequences: A case study on rural indigenous women in Bangladesh. *Australasian Journal of Regional Studies, 20*(2), 351.

Uddin, J., Hossin, M. Z., Mahbub, F., & Hossain, M. Z. (2013). Healthcare-seeking behavior among the Chakma ethnic group in Bangladesh: Can accessibility and cultural beliefs shape healthcare utilization? *International Quarterly of Community Health Education, 33*(4), 375–389. https://doi.org/10.2190/IQ.33.4.e

UN Women. (2020). *Intersectional feminism: What it means and why it matters right now*. Retrieved November 15, 2022, from https://www.unwomen.org/en/news/stories/2020/6/explainer-intersectiona-feminism-what-it-means-and-why-it-matters

CHAPTER 4

Healthcare on the Margins: Santal Women's Access Through an Intersectional Lens

Abstract This chapter evaluates different parameters of Santal women's access to public healthcare services during the COVID-19 outbreak from an intersectional perspective. To analyze the data, access to healthcare is evaluated by considering certain factors of accessibility. In this chapter, the healthcare-seeking of Santal women has been analyzed by measuring several factors, including their frequency of visiting public healthcare facilities, their preferred healthcare distinction, the role of education, stigma, and trust in healthcare-seeking, changes in healthcare-seeking behavior amid COVID-19, and vaccination acceptance among them. By comparing Santal women's health behavior and healthcare accessibility with that of Santal men and non-ethnic women, this chapter highlights the critical role of intersectional identity factors on women's access to healthcare services.

Keywords Healthcare access • Santal women • Awareness • Health-seeking behavior • COVID-19

The COVID-19 pandemic has exposed disparities in social determinants of health, leading to significant inequalities in COVID-19 health outcomes among different population groups. Furthermore, the pandemic's broader impacts have disproportionately affected social determinants of health, exacerbating health inequities (WHO, 2021). This is equally true for Bangladesh, as despite being the main recipients of Upazila Health

F. Nawaz, AN Bushra, *Santal Women and the Health Care Regime*, https://doi.org/10.1007/978-3-031-48872-6_4
51

Complex (UHC) provided healthcare services, healthcare access by women remained significantly low in Bangladesh. Women and children are the main recipients of UHC services (Mannan, 2013). However, ethnic women's access to healthcare services remains significantly poorer than that of ethnic men and non-ethnic women. The situation deteriorated as a global pandemic unfolded itself, disproportionately affecting different gender and ethnic groups (IISD, 2021; Sarker et al., 2023). When considering women's access to health, it is important to look at women's access to and control over resources and how they perceive their healthcare needs. It is also worthwhile to consider the environmental context, which is the social reality in a patriarchal society like Bangladesh, where the social structure is generally in favor of males and under their control. To explore the access to healthcare services of rural tribal women, such as Santal women, two questions were important to consider: what determines access to health services? And how? The following section of this chapter attempts to answer these two questions.

Access to Healthcare: To What Extent and How?

To comprehensively examine accessibility factors, it is imperative to first delve into the respondents' visitation patterns to healthcare facilities, encompassing both the public and private sectors. The Santal community, in particular, has demonstrated limited awareness and commitment to their healthcare requirements. The ensuing table illuminates the frequency with which the study participants sought healthcare services (Table 4.1).

Table 4.1 Santal women's frequency of visiting healthcare facilities during COVID-19

Number of times visiting a healthcare facility	Number and percentage of Santal women	
	UHC	Private facility
Never	12 (30%)	4 (10%)
Once or twice	22 (55%)	12 (30%)
Several times	2 (5%)	20 (50%)
Always	4 (10%)	4 (10%)
Total	40 (100%)	40 (100%)

Source: Field data

The primary data reveals a concerning trend among Santal women regarding their utilization of public healthcare facilities for seeking healthcare. Of the Santal women surveyed, 30% stated that they never visited the UHC during the coronavirus outbreak, compared to only 10% who never visited private healthcare facilities. Additionally, 55% of the respondents reported visiting UHC once or twice during the pandemic, while the same number (30%) visited private healthcare facilities once or twice. Further analysis shows that 50% of the respondents visited private healthcare facilities several times, whereas only 5% reported multiple visits to the UHC. Surprisingly, 10% of the respondents considered UHC as their primary healthcare facility, which is the same percentage as those who preferred private health facilities. These findings suggest a shift in Santal women's trust toward private healthcare facilities, as a larger percentage of them visited UHC only once or twice compared to private facilities. However, the situation changes drastically when it comes to multiple visits, with a significant difference between the percentages of Santals visiting private healthcare facilities multiple times (50%) versus those visiting UHC (5%).

An intriguing observation from the aforementioned table merits attention. It reveals a rise in the number of Santal women who accessed private healthcare services on multiple occasions compared to those who used private health services only once. Notably, a significant decrease occurred in the proportion of Santal women (10%) who consistently chose private healthcare facilities, as opposed to a higher percentage (50%) who visited these facilities several times. This data suggests that Santal women have positive experiences and confidence in private healthcare services, motivating them to prefer private hospitals over the UHC. As evidenced by the majority of respondents (20, representing 50% of Santal women in this study) revisiting private hospitals on multiple occasions, their favorable experiences have influenced their choices. However, it is worth noting that a mere 10% of respondents stated that they exclusively seek private healthcare, indicating that despite their trust and positive encounters with private health services, only a small fraction of Santal women can afford continuous reliance on private hospitals.

The data regarding Santal women seeking healthcare from the UHC versus private healthcare reveals significant disparities. Among the respondents, 55% reported visiting the UHC once or twice during the coronavirus pandemic. However, this number notably decreased, with only 10% of Santal women visiting the UHC on every healthcare occasion and 5%

going there occasionally but not always. The data highlights that the majority of Santal women visited the UHC once or twice and are unlikely to return for further treatment, as only 5% reported multiple visits and 10% consistently chose the UHC for treatment, showing a significant drop from the one-time users' data. The study's respondents indicated several key reasons for this change in attitude toward the UHC, including poor behavior of health providers, a lack of trust in UHC services, and negative past experiences. Despite their financial constraints as predominantly poor individuals, the Santals still tend to prefer private healthcare facilities over the UHC for their healthcare needs. They are even willing to take out loans and sell assets to access private healthcare services.

Existing studies support this finding as well. Alam et al. (2021), for instance, have argued that people have greater confidence in the private sector's responses to the COVID-19 virus compared to the GoB's preparedness efforts. This lack of trust in public health institutions and response to COVID-19 is found to hinder care-seeking (Joarder et al., 2020). The skepticism in the Nachol Upazila Health Complex (NUHC) is rooted in perceived inefficiency, negative perceptions, and discriminatory behavior within the institution. Similar findings from studies on the health-seeking behavior of tribal communities in Bangladesh align with this preference for private healthcare, as they also exhibit a preference for private healthcare due to perceived irregularities, misbehavior, and doctor unavailability in public health facilities. Interestingly, this pattern of preferring private healthcare services is not exclusive to ethnic patients, as non-ethnic patients have shown similar inclination toward private healthcare during the COVID-19 pandemic (Islam et al., 2019; Mohiuddin, 2020).

The discussion and data presented above highlight a clear trend among Santal women. Those who possess the financial means and opportunities tend to opt for private healthcare services rather than seeking essential healthcare from the NUHC. However, the majority of Santal women, who are economically disadvantaged, have no other healthcare options but to rely on the NUHC. Despite the NUHC offering relatively affordable healthcare services, these costs can still be burdensome for them compared to their non-ethnic counterparts. Additionally, the intertwining of their ethnic and gender identities exposes Santal women to severe criticism and dishonorable comments from health providers at the NUHC. These factors collectively contribute to shaping their healthcare perceptions and priorities. Due to negative past experiences at the NUHC, their level of trust in public healthcare institutions is poor. As a result, they show a strong inclination to seek healthcare from private facilities, even when it imposes a significant financial strain on them.

Access to Healthcare Across Gender and Ethnicity

People come together based on their commonality. Several aspects of the lives of the non-ethnic poor and the poor Santals were similar. These similarities play a key role in building bridges between the acutely poor people of both groups. For instance, women belonging to both the Santal tribe and the non-ethnic communities lack ownership of resources, are married off and conceive their first child at a very young age, are less likely to educate themselves, and cannot afford quality healthcare. However, non-ethnic women do not work hard in the agricultural field with their men during their pregnancy like ethnic women frequently do. Non-ethnic women are also more likely to seek healthcare during pregnancy than ethnic women. Their experiences of disadvantage and discrimination unite them, but when the socio-cultural realities of each society are considered, the ethnic women turn out to be in a more unfavorable position. The following table compares the frequency of seeking healthcare by Santal women, Santal men, and non-ethnic women.

Table 4.2 makes a comparison of the frequency of seeking healthcare between Santal women, Santal men, and non-ethnic women. The proclivity of non-ethnic women to seek private healthcare is significantly higher than that of Santal women. Twenty-eight (70%) non-ethnic women interviewed in this study have expressed that they always go to private healthcare facilities for treatment, and 12 (30%) of non-ethnic women reported visiting private healthcare facilities several times in their lives. These numbers for ethnic women stand at 4 (10%) and 20 (50%), respectively. Twelve (30%) of the non-ethnic women had never visited NUHC in their lifetime, while the number remained the same for Santal women. Although the percentage is equal, the reasons for not visiting NUHC are different for these two groups. Non-ethnic women did not seek healthcare from the NUHC because they could afford private healthcare and preferred private healthcare services. On the contrary, Santal women who did not visit the NUHC even once are not able to afford even the cheap transportation and treatment costs at the NUHC, let alone at a private healthcare facility. Other dominant reasons for ethnic women not going to the NUHC are related to their health beliefs and the behavior of health providers.

Table 4.2   Frequency of seeking healthcare across gender and ethnic groups during COVID-19

Number of times visiting a healthcare facility	Number and percentage of Santal women		Number and percentage of Santal men		Number and percentage of non-ethnic rural women	
	UHC	Private facility	UHC	Private facility	UHC	Private facility
Never	12 (30%)	4 (10%)	27 (67.5%)	–	12 (30%)	–
Once or twice	22 (55%)	12 (30%)	13 (32.5%)	27 (67.5%)	12 (30%)	–
Several times	2 (5%)	20 (50%)	–	–	16 (40%)	12 (30%)
Always	4 (10%)	4 (10%)	–	13 (32.5%)	–	28 (70%)
Total	40 (100%)	40 (100%)	40 (100%)	40 (100%)	40 (100%)	40 (100%)

Source: Field research

The ratio of Santal men visiting the NUHC is comparatively lower than that of Santal women. The male members of the Santal community have a higher proportion of access to private healthcare services than the Santal women. All 40 (100%) Santal men interviewed had reported seeking private healthcare at some point in their lives. For 13 (32.5%) respondents, private hospitals are the go-to healthcare facility, and the other 27 (67.5%) have visited private hospitals once or twice in their lives. One reason behind it is that the Santal men enjoy better mobility than the Santal women. Most of the Santal women interviewed in this study have reported that they have never visited any place outside their village in their whole lives. Some of the Santal men own bicycles that allow them to visit private doctors away from home. Another reason is that the frequency of Santal men getting sick is significantly lower than that of Santal women. So, they (Santal men) seldom feel the need to see a doctor. Lesser incidents of sickness mean lower healthcare costs. So, the Santal men tend to pay more for better-quality healthcare. They simply cannot do it for their women, for they get sick frequently, and private healthcare costs for such frequent treatment would be devastating for poor Santal families.

Field investigations of this study have revealed that the general poor class of the locality is a victim of the unequal treatment of the UHC health providers, along with the Santal women, who are doubly disadvantaged due to their intersectional identity. The irregularities in the health delivery system, like preferential treatment, have decreased the confidence of the people in the services and impartiality of the NUHC. However, whereas non-ethnic people are sometimes seen to protest against the institutional irregularities that limit their access to healthcare services, Santal women are less likely to protest. This is because of the poor self-image they have. Years of unequal treatment by society have normalized the discriminatory treatment toward the Santals, and they have subconsciously accepted some of these discriminations as the norm or their fate. Such faiths have led them not to protest against institutional irregularities. Lower levels of education and awareness have a role to play here as well.

In this regard, one of the Santal women has asserted:

The locally influential people, who have a good relationship with the health providers of the UHC, get notified about the medicines when they arrive in stock, but we have to go through the process, often to hear that medicines are out of supply. The doctors and officials of the UHC are often absent as well, just like the medicines in stock. During the Corona vaccination campaign, some of our men protested against the volunteers who were working on behalf of the NUHC. NUHC volunteers were favoring their people even though we were standing before them in line for vaccines. The police punished our men, not the volunteers. We are disadvantaged everywhere, and we have no place to go. Taking a stand against irregularities only costs us but never solves our issues. Government hospitals are meant to provide healthcare to poor people. But if the authorities keep manipulating the system to benefit the people closer to them, where would we poor people go? (FGD on October 20, 2022)

One of the doctors at the NUHC confirmed the claim made by Santal women about the preferential treatment being given by health providers at the NUHC to the local elite and influential people. However, according to this doctor, it is necessary to keep a good relationship with the locals to operate here without any hassle. The doctor has asserted:

Operating in a rural area is not an easy task. We are always in danger because you never know when the local goons and politically powerful people will come and attack us for no reason. During our coronavirus vaccination programs, we had to handle a lot of unwanted situations where illegal benefits were claimed by the local powerholders and politicians. They are always ready to attack the hospital and its property, even the doctors. We have to handle them carefully.

The Santals are not like this… It's for our own safety that we allow some extra benefits to the local elites. We need their support; that's why. (In-depth interview with NHCD-1 on October 20, 2022)

This narrative illustrates the underlying presence of unequal treatment, nepotism, and favoritism within NUHC toward its service recipients. Such behavior from healthcare providers erodes people's trust in the institution and its services, ultimately hindering accessibility. Particularly, the preferential treatment given to influential local individuals by UHC health providers has been a significant factor limiting the healthcare accessibility of impoverished Santal women. Curiously, this issue remains absent from the existing scholarly works on UHC healthcare services. The assertions made in the aforementioned story find support in additional evidence documented in local and national daily newspapers. As highlighted by Zohir (2021), instances of nepotism, preferential treatment, and harassment of NUHC service recipients during a vaccination campaign resulted in a negative response, leading to the imposition of fines on the recipients. The complexities surrounding these dynamics further accentuate the perplexities encountered in addressing healthcare disparities and inequities within the institution.

Other research on the healthcare access of the ethnic population in Bangladesh has also revealed irregularities and nepotism in public healthcare facilities. Seddiky (2020), in his study on community clinics, has illuminated the fact that nepotism is prevalent in community clinics' service provision. Affluent and influential patients with higher education and social status receive preferential treatment. They are provided with extensive medication, including antibiotics and contraceptives for their family members, by Community Healthcare Providers (CHCPs). In contrast, day laborers and migrant patients face obstacles in accessing medication due to perceived reluctance from healthcare providers, which is linked to their lack of regional residency documentation (Seddiky, 2020). This is equally true for developed countries, as Chen et al. (2021) express that in the USA, structural inequalities during the pandemic have exacerbated healthcare access barriers, particularly for low-income individuals and people of color who face heightened health risks, transportation access difficulties, and increased economic hardships due to COVID-19.

HEALTH LITERACY, STIGMA, AND FEAR

Lower levels of education contribute to susceptibility to misinformation, while trust and stigma can influence information-seeking behaviors and attitudes toward healthcare systems. The illiteracy of the ethnic minority communities in Bangladesh made them vulnerable to fake news and misconceptions about the pandemic (Kabir, 2020). Education levels are notably low among minority ethnic groups, with only 9% literacy and 2% having completed secondary education (cited in Alam, 2022). As a result, the majority of them work as day laborers. Indigenous rights groups, including the Bangladesh Adivasi Forum (BAF), Jatiya Adivasi Parishad (JAP), and Kapaeeng Foundation, reported that approximately 90% of indigenous people in rural areas worked as day laborers and lost their income due to the pandemic (cited in Rozario, 2020). Existing studies show that excessive media coverage of lockdowns, quarantines, and social distancing measures contributed to the spread of rumors, particularly affecting vulnerable groups such as low-income individuals, female workers, and healthcare employees (Mahmud et al., 2022). Santal women, who had reportedly lost their income in COVID-19, have shown a higher inclination toward misinformation, COVID-19-related stigma, and a lower level of trust in healthcare providers and the COVID-19 management strategies of the government.

Table 4.3 illustrates the educational levels of Santal women. Among the Santal women, the majority (50%) were illiterate, while 35% had completed primary education, enabling them to read, write, and sign names. Some of the illiterate Santal women had attended primary school but remained unable to read, write, or sign names. Only a small proportion of

Table 4.3 Average level of education of the respondents

Average level of education	Santal women
Fully illiterate	20 (50%)
Primary level	14 (35%)
Secondary level (SSC)	4 (10%)
Higher Secondary level (HSC)	2 (5%)
Total	40 (100%)

Source: Field research

Santal women (5%) completed the HSC level, and 10% completed the SSC level. In this study, the average educational attainment of Santal women slightly exceeded that of Santal men. However, the field investigation suggests that gender and education level play minimal or almost no role in the Santals' perception, trust, and stigmatization of COVID-19.

One of the respondents to this study has reported that:

One of the hardest parts for me was the stigma that came with COVID-19. People in our village started to view anyone who got sick as if they had done something wrong. It was as if we were being blamed for our own misfortune. The fear and mistrust in our community grew, and many began avoiding those who were affected, including me. I fell ill with symptoms that felt like a cold, but I was too afraid to tell anyone. The stigma surrounding the virus made it seem like a shameful thing to admit. I kept my symptoms a secret, hoping they would go away on their own. I didn't want my family to be subjected to the same stigma I had witnessed others endure. In time, my condition worsened, and I had no choice but to seek medical help. The journey to the nearest health-care center was long and difficult. and the discrimination I faced there was disheartening. However, the treatment I received from my peers seemed worse. (EWL-8, in-depth interview on November 2, 2022)

Another respondent has reported:

For generations, we have followed our own spiritual practices, seeking blessings and guidance from our deities and ancestors. But during the COVID-19 lock-down, it was hard for us to gather together and perform religious activities to seek blessings from our ancestors. I had no choice but to believe the information provided by the government and NGOs. But I couldn't read the information pamphlets or understand the nature of the virus. So, my primary information source was the chatting I do with my neighbors and friends. They would share with me things they had heard about the virus from TV news and other community members. But the fear of the unknown persisted within me. What if we get affected? What if vaccination brought harm instead of protection? With the support and encouragement of the community health workers and NGO professionals I trusted, I eventually overcame my fear and got vaccinated. (EWL-6, in-depth interview on November 2, 2022)

The field investigation of this study has revealed another interesting thing. While the health-seeking behavior and stigma of the non-ethnic women were driven by a lack of trust in the public declaration and the government information source, Santal women were more motivated by religious faith, illiteracy, and fear. Moreover, the pre-existing lack of trust in NUHC health providers and health services also made Santal women not to seek treatment amidst the COVID-19 outbreak. Contrary to what was established by Mahmud et al. (2022), vulnerable groups such as low-income individuals and female workers in the Santal community were not the most vulnerable to COVID-19-related rumors and stigma. The field investigation of the present study revealed that, although Santal women were exposed to COVID-19-related misinformation, had lower levels of education, and had financial uncertainty, they were more likely to trust the government vaccination campaigns during the pandemic. NGOs have played a significant awareness-building role in this regard. More details on this issue will be discussed in the following section.

Adapting to the New Normal Amidst COVID-19

Among the many negative effects of the COVID-19 virus, there are some positive ones as well. In the field investigation, it was observed that the virus outbreak caused behavioral changes among the study respondents. This positive behavioral change has the potential to improve their collective health status. And if not directly, it can have an indirect but greater impact on the Santal women's access to healthcare. The aspects of behavior that were changed during the pandemic on a large scale are cleanliness, food habits, and healthcare awareness. Some respondents have reported no change in behavior as well, but the ratio is insignificant compared to those who have developed healthy habits.

Table 4.4 shows that four (10%) Santal women have reported experiencing no behavioral change after the pandemic. Twenty-two (55%) of the Santal women have reported that they are practicing cleanliness after the coronavirus. The practice of cleanliness involves personal hygiene, keeping the living space clean and healthy, washing hands with cleaning substances, washing hands after the toilet and before eating, and using clean and safe water. None of the Santal women and men have reported following social distancing measures and reducing the frequent visits to their neighbors. Thirty-two (80%) of the Santal women have reported using masks during the pandemic, whereas none of the Santal men interviewed have done so. The proportion of Santal women using masks is greater than that of non-ethnic women, as found in the field investigation. This higher proportion of masks used by Santal women is also a result of free mask distribution

Table 4.4 COVID-19-
induced behavioral change

Behavior	Santal women
No change	4 (10%)
Cleanliness	22 (55%)
Using masks	32 (80%)
Increased awareness	6 (15%)
Food habit change	18 (45%)
Total	40 (100%)

Source: Field research

and awareness campaigns in Santal villages by NGOs operating in the localities.

Among all other COVID-19-induced behavioral changes, increased healthcare awareness and changes in food habits are probably the most important ones. Six (15%) of the Santal women interviewed in this study have reported that after COVID-19 they are now more aware and sincere about their healthcare needs than before. They are now more likely to seek healthcare for issues that they were likely to ignore before the pandemic outbreak. This positive attitude has the potential to enhance health perception and healthcare needs in the coming days. Eighteen (45%) of the Santal women have reported a change in their food habits. The reasons that led to this change are twofold. One is due to income loss and other economic crises; the Santal women had decreased their food intake. The second reason is that, because of the pandemic, some Santal women have become aware of the importance of eating clean and healthy foods and are likely to avoid foods that have negative health effects.

One of the respondents asserted that:

> *Before the coronavirus, I had never thought that a simple cough and fever could be so deadly. Every day, the TV news reported that a lot of people were dying. I also get colds and fevers sometimes. But I never thought that it was something worth seeking treatment for. I don't even take medicine for my menstrual belly ache. But as I have seen a lot of posters, TV advertisements, and COVID-19-related programs, I have realized that no symptoms should be taken lightly. Since the virus outbreak, I regularly wash my hands with soap, use clean water, and try to remain as clean as possible.* (EWL-7, in-depth interview on November 2, 2022)

The field investigations suggest that the pandemic outbreak has made the Santal women more aware. Lack of awareness and negligence in healthcare are major barriers to accessing healthcare. Increased awareness means a positive change in the attitude and health-seeking behavior of the Santal women. The increased awareness is a result of the awareness-building activities, programs, posters, and advertisements by the NGOs and NHUC. Although, initially, the Santal women were aware of cleanliness and the protective measures of the coronavirus, a significant shift is taking place in their healthcare-seeking attitude as they are now recognizing and prioritizing their healthcare needs.

Some of the pre-COVID-19 studies on the public health of ethnic communities have argued that there is unequal access to water, sanitation, and hygiene (WASH) services between minority ethnic groups (residing in the Chittagong Hill Tracts (CHT) region) and the Bengali population in Bangladesh. This disparity stems from a complex interplay of micro-level systems, social factors, institutions, ideologies, policies, and processes that collectively perpetuate injustice against minority communities (Alam, 2022). Our findings from Santal Polli of Nachol, however, suggest that ethnic people of the plains enjoy comparatively better access to water, sanitation, and hygiene than those living in the CHT area. The awareness-building measures taken during and post-COVID-19 have raised awareness regarding hygiene, water, and sanitation (Fig. 4.1).

Vaccination and Health Consciousness

This study explored some of the root causes that shape the health perceptions of the Santal women, as it is a significant determinant of their health-seeking behavior, which ultimately guides their accessibility to preferred healthcare options. The field investigation reveals that Santal women rarely recognize their healthcare needs. Recognizing healthcare needs is a prerequisite for seeking care. This negligence is a result of a combination of factors, including financial affordability, a lack of education and awareness, poor healthcare literacy, a lack of information, and health perception. These factors, in the first place, determine whether the Santal women will consider taking treatment for a health issue or ignore their healthcare needs. The previous encounters of the Santal women with the NUHC have discouraged them from considering visiting the facility again. As long as they could afford private healthcare, Santal women tended to avoid

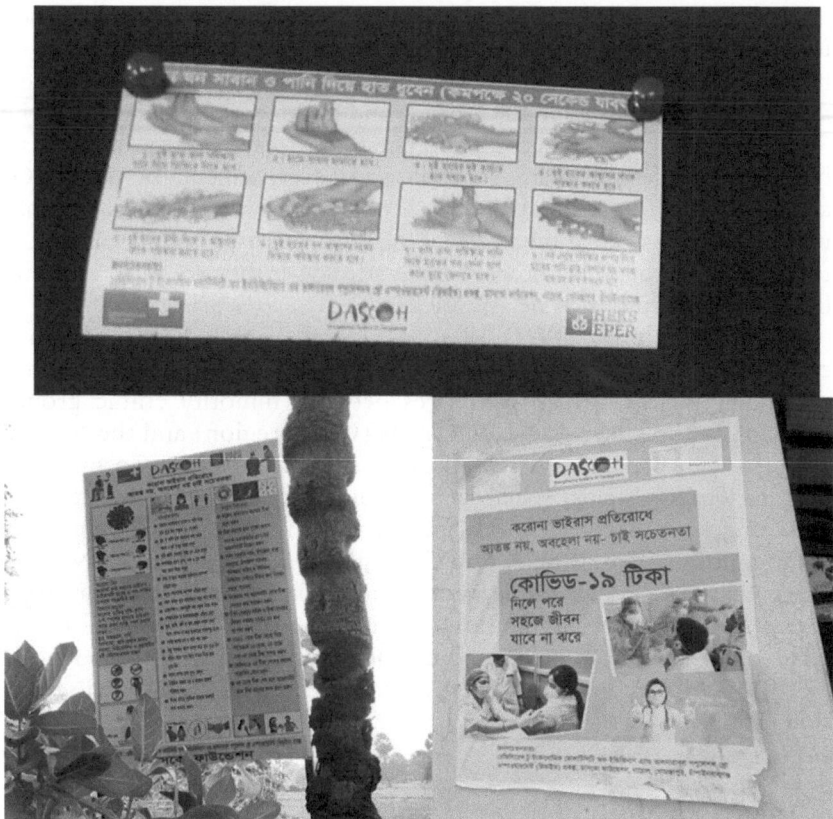

Fig. 4.1 COVID-19 awareness-building posters in Santal villages by DASCOH foundation

NUHC services. However, an unfortunate reality is that the majority of Santal families are financially unable to visit private healthcare facilities. So, on many occasions, they ignore healthcare needs to avoid visiting the NUHC (Fig. 4.2).

Even though the Santal women have an overall negative perception of the NUHC services, their participation in the COVID-19 vaccination program shows otherwise. The rate of COVID-19 vaccination is quite high among Santal women. One of the noteworthy factors behind this development is that the NUHC played an amazing role in COVID-19

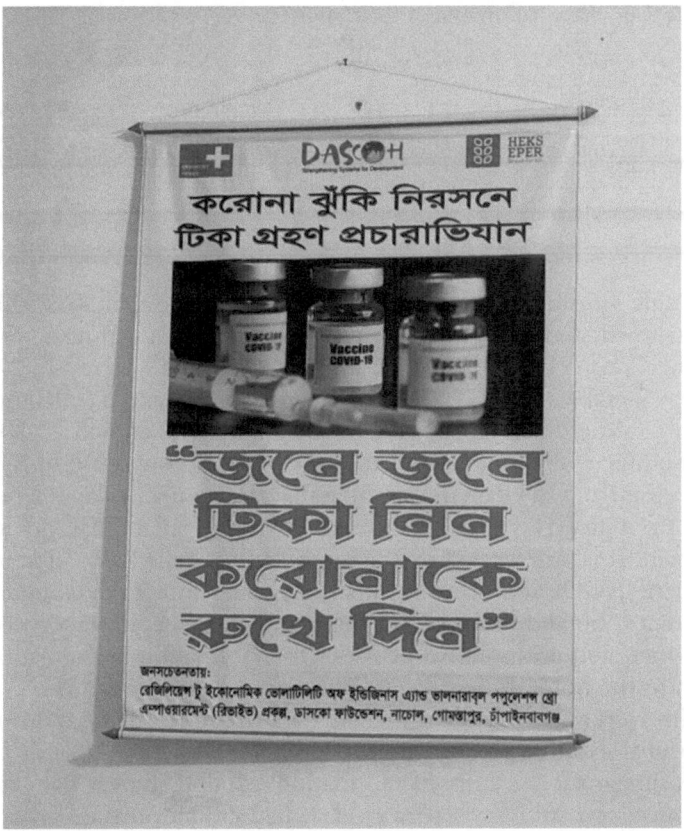

Fig. 4.2 COVID-19 vaccination awareness efforts by DASCOH foundation

crisis management. Along with the NUHC, some local voluntary organizations and NGOs also contributed to the awareness building, information dissemination, and vaccination campaign of the NUHC. The officials of the NUHC collected COVID-19 samples from the root level through the community clinics. In a word, both institutional and community actors came together during the coronavirus crisis to tackle the unimaginable situation. As a result of the combined efforts by the NUHC and other community actors, the NUHC has so far been successful in providing vaccines to the maximum number of people in the area.

Table 4.5 Vaccination rate of the respondents

Doses of vaccine	Santal women	Santal men	Non-ethnic women
First dose	34 (85%)	40 (100%)	32 (80%)
Second dose	27 (67.5%)	40 (100%)	24 (60%)
Booster dose	11 (27.5%)	8 (20%)	8 (20%)

Source: Field research

Table 4.5 shows that 34 (85%) of the Santal women, 40 (100%) of the Santal men, and 8 (80%) of the non-ethnic women had taken the first jab of the Corona vaccine. The second dose was administered to 27 (67.5%) of the Santal women, 3 (100%) of the Santal men, and 6 (60%) of the non-ethnic women. Eleven (27.5%) of the Santal women and 2 (20%) of the non-ethnic women have reported taking the booster dose of the vaccine. It is clear from the data in this table that the number of Santal people taking the COVID-19 vaccine is a little higher than that of non-ethnic women. It is, as revealed by the respondents of the study, due to the fact that the NGOs and other voluntary organizations have conducted more awareness-building campaigns, mask and cleaning substance distribution activities, and promotional activities for vaccination in the Santal villages than in the non-ethnic villages. The respondents have also reported that health workers have visited their houses to inform them about the safety measures required to survive the pandemic (Fig. 4.3).

A similar success story of vaccination is found all over Bangladesh. For instance, one study by Savira et al. (2022) found in their cross-sectional study that the COVID-19 vaccine acceptance rate is very high in rural Bangladesh (95%). The Bangladeshi government's adept use of diplomatic and health strategies, built upon a track record of successful vaccination campaigns and prior experience, enabled them to effectively tackle the COVID-19 pandemic. Their proactive approach led to a quicker flattening of the infection curve compared to many developed nations, allowing for a gradual return to normalcy in society and the economy (Nazmunnahar et al., 2023). Due to the smart and timely efforts by the Government of Bangladesh (GoB), more than 250 million vaccine doses have been given, and over 115 million individuals in the country have received both doses of the vaccine by May 2022 (UNICEF, 2022). Thus, the higher degree of vaccination among the Santal community living in rural Bangladesh is no surprise at all.

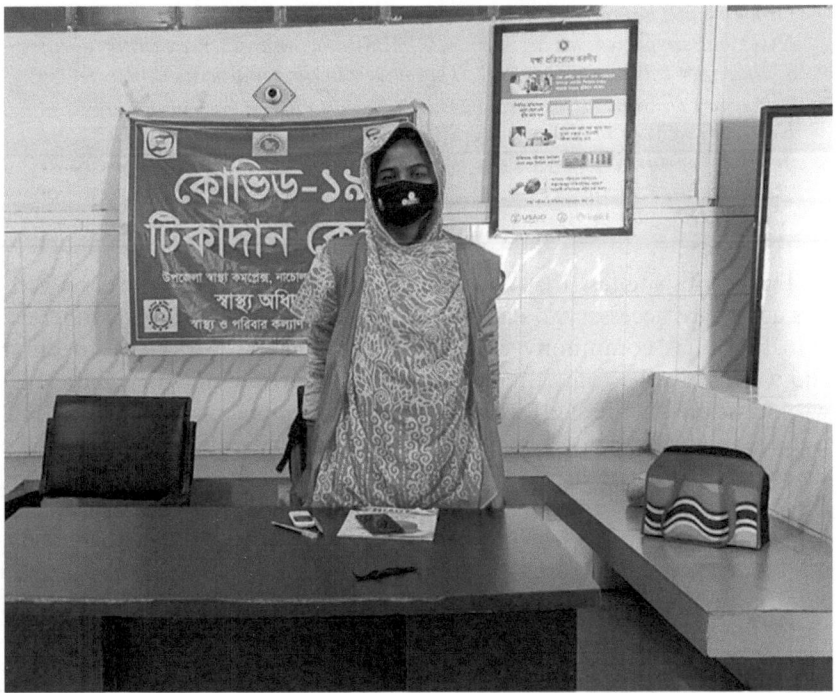

Fig. 4.3 COVID-19 vaccination corner at the NUHC

One respondent to this study has reported:

I have taken two jabs of Corona vaccines. We collected our **Tika card** *(an online registration card for taking vaccines) from a local computer shop. Then we had to go to a nearby school to get the vaccine. A number of NGOs, along with NUHC health workers, have visited our village several times during the coronavirus. The DASCOH Foundation and Ashroy have distributed masks and soaps and told us why taking the vaccine and maintaining social distancing are necessary. They have been very active with these awareness-building measures. The NUHC often announces necessary health-related information using loudspeakers throughout the community. Everyone was very helpful. When the time comes, I will take the booster dose as well.* (EWL-8, in-depth interview on November 2, 2022)

Another Santal woman has reported that:

I am a member of the DASCOH NGO. During the coronavirus pandemic, my NGO has supported me with masks, handwash, and other cleaning agents because they want us to stay safe. They have distributed several leaflets in our village as well, which showcase how to wash hands during the Corona outbreak. Now I try to wash my hands accordingly and follow whatever the NGO people instruct. No one from my village has the virus. I think following these cleanliness measures could be a reason. (EWL-4, in-depth interview on November 2, 2022)

The stories suggest that concentrated and cooperative efforts by various actors are necessary to deal with a public health crisis like a pandemic. If institutional, community, and non-governmental actors come together and work toward a common objective, they can overcome their individual weaknesses and achieve greater success. The attempts made by the NUHC were praiseworthy, but a number of shortcomings of the NUCH have always posed a barrier to accessing healthcare for Santal women. However, a cooperative and organized effort, including both the community and other public health actors, has helped them overcome their institutional limitations and reach a greater number of people with their public healthcare programs. In the case of COVID-19 crisis management, the local NGOs had provided better knowledge about the Santals and procured additional funding from their donors to distribute masks and build awareness, and the local volunteers had filled the human resource gap of the NUHC.

CONCLUSION

In this chapter, the knowledge and awareness factors of healthcare accessibility among Santal women have been analyzed through an intersectional lens. The findings of this chapter report that the frequency of health-seeking among Santal women is very low in comparison to that of ethnic men and non-ethnic women. This health behavior is shaped by a low level of education and a high level of exposure to social stigma, poor perception and experience of NUHC services, low affordability of healthcare, poor digital literacy and technical support, and finally, a lack of awareness about healthcare needs. Education attainment does not have a positive correlation with the healthcare accessibility of Santal women, as it neither uplifts their socio-economic status nor improves their healthcare awareness. The COVID-19 pandemic, however, has caused a positive change in the healthcare awareness of Santal women, despite a significant institutional deficiency in the healthcare system. Cooperative efforts by different healthcare providers to manage public health during the pandemic have played a crucial role in the growing healthcare awareness of Santal women.

References

Alam, E., Al Abdouli, K., Khamis, A. H., Bhuiyan, H. U., & Rahman, K. A. (2021). Public trust in COVID-19 prevention and responses between January and May 2020 in Bangladesh. *Risk Management and Healthcare Policy, 14*, 4425–4437.

Alam, M. Z. (2022). Ethnic inequalities in access to WASH in Bangladesh. *The Lancet Global Health, 10*(8), E1086–E1087. https://doi.org/10.1016/S2214-109X(22)00232-7

Chen, K. L., Brozen, M., Rollman, J. E., Ward, T., Norris, K. C., Gregory, K. D., & Zimmerman, F. J. (2021). How is the COVID-19 pandemic shaping transportation access to health care? *Transportation Research Interdisciplinary Perspectives, 10*, 100338. https://doi.org/10.1016/j.trip.2021.100338

IISD. (2021, August 31). COVID-19 wreaking havoc on Bangladesh's poor: A story of food, cash, and health crises. Retrieved October 10, 2023, from https://sdg.iisd.org/commentary/guest-articles/covid-19-wreaking-havoc-on-bangladeshs-poor-a-story-of-food-cash-and-health-crises/

Islam, M. Z., Zaman, F., Farjana, S., & Khanam, S. (2019). Accessibility to health care services of Upazila Health Complex: Experience of rural people. *Journal of Preventive and Social Medicine, 38*(2), 30–37.

Joarder, T., Bin Khaled, M. N., & Zaman, S. (2020, December 3). Trust in the Bangladeshi health system during the COVID-19 pandemic: A mixed-methods exploration (Version 1) [Preprint]. *Research Square.* https://doi.org/10.21203/rs.3.rs-117196/v1

Kabir, M. M. (2020, August 11). Life and livelihood crisis of ethnic minorities in the Covid-19 pandemic. *The Business Standard.* https://www.tbsnews.net/thoughts/life-and-livelihoods-crisis-ethnic-minorities-covid-19-pandemic-118111%3famp

Mahmud, A., Zaman, F., & Islam, M. R. (2022). COVID-19 syndemic, stigmatization, and social vulnerabilities: A case of Bangladesh. *Local Development & Society, 2*, 242–266. https://doi.org/10.1080/26883597.2021.1952846

Mannan, M. A. (2013). Access to public health facilities in Bangladesh: A study on facility utilisation and burden of treatment. *The Bangladesh Development Studies, 36*(4).

Mohiuddin, A. K. (2020). Patient satisfaction with healthcare services: Bangladesh perspective. *International Journal of Public Health Science, 9*(1), 34–45.

Nazmunnahar, A. B., Haque, M. A., Tanbir, M., Roknuzzaman, A. S. M., Sarker, R., & Rabiul Islam, M. (2023). COVID-19 vaccination success in Bangladesh: Key strategies were prompt response, early drives for vaccines, and effective awareness campaigns. *Health Science Reports, 6*(5), e1281. https://doi.org/10.1002/hsr2.1281

Rozario, S. U. (2020, April 20). Ethnic communities face starvation in Bangladesh. *UCA News.* Retrieved October 5, 2023, from https://www.ucanews.com/amp/ethnic-communities-face-starvation-in-bangladesh/87768

Sarker, M. R., Sarkar, M. A. R., Alam, M. J., Begum, I. A., & Bhandari, H. (2023). Systems thinking on the gendered impacts of COVID-19 in Bangladesh: A systematic review. *Heliyon, 9*(2), e13773. https://doi.org/10.1016/j.heliyon.2023.e13773

Savira, F., Alif, S. M., Afroz, A., Siddiquea, B. N., Shetty, A., Chowdhury, H. A., Bhattacharya, O., Khan Chowdhury, M. R., Islam, M. S., Ali, L., & Billah, B. (2022). Evaluation of COVID-19 vaccine acceptance and uptake in rural Bangladesh: A cross-sectional study. *BMJ Open, 12*(12), e064468. https://doi.org/10.1136/bmjopen-2022-064468

Seddiky, M. A. (2020). Decentralized health service delivery system in Bangladesh: Evaluating community clinics in promoting healthcare for the rural poor. *European Scientific Journal, 16*(12), 253. https://doi.org/10.19044/esj.2020.v16n12p253

UNICEF. (2022, May 31). *Bangladesh's COVID-19 vaccination rate has soared in a year.* UNICEF. Retrieved September 29, 2023, from https://www.unicef.org/stories/bangladesh-covid-19-vaccination-rate-has-soared

World Health Organization. (2021). COVID-19 and the social determinants of health and health equity: Evidence brief. Retrieved October 10, 2023, from https://iris.who.int/bitstream/handle/10665/348333/9789240038387-eng.pdf

Zohir, Z. I. (2021, August 18). Nachole corona tika nite asa seba grohitake orthodondo. *Mahananda TV.* Retrieved December 21, 2022, from https://cutt.ly/X0Ml246

CHAPTER 5

Unveiling Santal Women's Healthcare Challenges During the Pandemic

Abstract This chapter explores the challenges experienced by Santal women in accessing healthcare services during the pandemic. In this chapter, all challenges are organized into four broad groups, including the personal and behavioral challenges of Santal women determining their health-seeking behavior and access to health, institutional challenges, financial challenges, and challenges in accessing telehealth services during the coronavirus outbreak. To provide a comprehensive understanding of Santal women's healthcare accessibility in Bangladesh, this chapter examines the challenges faced by both Santal women and healthcare providers.

Keywords Santal women • Institutional barriers • UHC • Health-seeking behavior

THE INSTITUTIONAL IMPEDIMENTS TO SANTAL WOMEN'S HEALTH

Santal women were victims of institutional challenges. These challenges hindered their access to healthcare. The major institutional challenges for the healthcare accessibility of Santal women included a shortage of medicines at the Upazila Health Complex (UHC) and the absenteeism of the health providers. These institutional challenges are supported by some of the limitations of the Nachol Upazila Health Complex (NUHC). The

F. Nawaz, AN Bushra, *Santal Women and the Health Care Regime*, https://doi.org/10.1007/978-3-031-48872-6_5

unequal attitude and behavior of the healthcare providers toward Santal women contribute to the institutional inefficiency in limiting their access to healthcare. The NUHC has undertaken some noteworthy steps to promote the health of the Santal women and overcome some of the institutional limitations. However, both the field investigation of this study and the existing scholarship have revealed these attempts to be ineffective.

Islam et al. (2020), for instance, suggest that a shortage of well-equipped hospitals, limited testing facilities, low awareness levels, inadequate knowledge, inconsistent adherence to safety measures, widespread poverty, and precarious employment conditions have contributed to the spread of COVID-19 in Bangladesh. Another study by Biswas et al. (2020) suggests that Bangladesh has faced significant challenges in preparing for and responding to the COVID-19 pandemic. These challenges have both short-term and long-term implications, affecting health, the economy, and governance. According to them, these challenges include a lack of planning and coordination, unequal resource allocation, strained healthcare infrastructure, bureaucratic delays, ineffective risk communication, leadership issues among authorities, and disjointed decision-making processes. These challenges have created a precarious situation with uncertain consequences for the future.

Table 5.1 unravels the factors behind respondents not choosing UHC as a healthcare destination by the respondents of this study.

In the interviews and FGDs, it was found that 18 (45%) of the Santal women and 14 (35%) Santal men have reported the discriminatory behavior of the health providers as their prime reason for not having confidence in the NUHC services. The non-ethnic women have also reported the discriminatory and preferential treatment of the health providers, but that did not keep them from accessing the health services from the NUHC. Six (15%) of Santal women, eight (20%) of Santal men, and eight (20%) of

Table 5.1 Major reasons for not choosing UHC as a healthcare destination

Reasons	Santal women	Santal men	Non-ethnic women
Discriminatory treatment	18 (45%)	14 (35%)	12 (30%)
Unavailability of doctors	6 (15%)	8 (20%)	8 (20%)
Unavailability of drugs	10 (25%)	10 (25%)	4 (10%)
Can afford private treatment	6 (15%)	8 (20%)	16 (40%)
Total	40 (100%)	40 (100%)	40 (100%)

Source: Field research

non-ethnic women have reported the unavailability of doctors as an issue. Ten (25%) of the Santal women, 10 (25%) of the Santal men, and 4 (10%) of the non-ethnic women have reported the unavailability of drugs as their leading reason for not choosing UHC as a healthcare option. Another 6 (15%) Santal women, 8 (20%) Santal men, and 16 (40%) non-ethnic women have expressed that they do not prefer UHC as a healthcare destination simply because they can afford private treatment. In the following section, the critical challenges of healthcare accessibility are explored further.

Missing from the Radar: Identifying the Invisible Vulnerable

One of the health providers of the NUHC interviewed in this study expressed her optimism and positive thoughts about the NUHC's role in promoting inclusivity in healthcare accessibility. The free medicine distribution, medical camps, and training sessions with the local people on healthcare awareness are some of the most significant attempts undertaken by the NUHC to include Santal women in their healthcare delivery system. Each month, two to four medical camps are arranged in the Santal villages, as well as in other remote areas. In these medical camps, treatments, training, and free medicines are distributed to the people. Free medicines are also distributed through community clinics. Along with these, a separate budget is kept to meet ethnic people's healthcare needs. However, the testimony of the respondents to the study does not fully agree with these claims of the NUHC professionals.

In this regard, one of the respondents has asserted that:

Nachol Upazila Health Complex has been a model for efficient service delivery. We have the highest number of Corona vaccinations, and our facility was not shut off for a single day during the pandemic. NUHC has a separate budget for the indigenous people of the locality. We use this budget to provide free medicines to them. We also arrange several medical camps for the Santal villages every now and then. In these medical camps, we teach the Santals healthy habits and healthcare awareness. Along with these medical camps, training sessions on menstrual hygiene and antenatal and postnatal care are organized for the Santal women. The one thing that is holding us back is that we do not have any surgeons here, and the security staff is not adequate in number. We try our best to reach all the people in this area. (KII-1, Key Informant Interview on October 20, 2022)

This expression discloses a number of aspects of the NUHC services that promote greater inclusion of Santal women. The field investigations of this study conform to the attempts of the NUHC to promote inclusivity in health service provision, as claimed by the NUHC health providers. However, all these attempts made by the NUHC did not actually benefit those who were the most vulnerable and deserving of these services. NUHC medical camps were found to be arranged in areas where the quality of life of Santal families was significantly better than that of most other Santals, who lead miserable lives. The people of Lakkhanpur village were in a much better position than the people of Hakroil village in terms of financial affordability, level of education and awareness, involvement with multiple income-generating activities, NGO presence, and availability of safe drinking water and proper sanitation. However, the people of Hakroil village have reported that the last UHC medical camp arranged in their village dates back a few years, whereas the respondents of Lakkhanpur have reported the frequent organization of medical camps in their locality. One of the NUHC service recipients has asserted:

> *The NUHC health providers had come to our village a few years ago when a diarrhea epidemic broke out in our village. Since then, no medical camp or such things have taken place in our village by the NUHC. Not even during the coronavirus outbreak. During the COVID-19 pandemic, some NGOs like DASCOH and Ashroy arranged meetings and camps where they distributed masks, and other equipment to fight Corona. They also talked about the benefits of keeping clean. But they had never provided us with free medicines, and so did the NUHC. NUHC has broadcast some corona-related information on loudspeakers. Apart from this, we didn't notice any medical camps, free medicine distributions, or other such things during the coronavirus pandemic. Santals, who have money and agricultural lands, get the benefits from government services, whereas we are largely overlooked by the authorities.* (FGD on October 20, 2022)

Although the respondents of Hakroil village have largely reported that there was no medical camp arranged in their village during the COVID-19 pandemic, the respondents of Lakkhanpur village have reported otherwise. The NUHC organized medical camps, which thus failed to benefit the most vulnerable portion of the study population. This inability to identify and prioritize the most vulnerable Santal women had created a situation where all the developmental efforts for Santals were directed toward villages where the Santals were in an overall better state comparatively, leaving the other Santal population in poverty and disadvantage. Twenty (50%) respondents to this study living in Hakroil village have reported being completely deprived of the benefits of the NUHC initiatives (medical camps and health awareness training sessions) that were meant to promote inclusivity in health service delivery. Those who have been beneficiaries of medical camps and other NUHC campaigns have reported minimal effects of these initiatives on their healthcare awareness and health-seeking behavior.

The Struggle with Medicine Scarcity

A shortage of medicines at the UHC dominates Santal women's choice of not choosing the UHC as their healthcare destination. Twenty-six (65%) of the Santal women and four (10%) non-ethnic women have reported that they do not go to the UHC due to the frequent unavailability of drugs. Even though the poor are entitled to free medicines from the UHC, they do not often get them as the health providers often report a shortage of medicines. As a result, the poor Santal women have to buy medicine from outside drug stores, which they can seldom afford. As they are not getting medicines from the UHC for free and are ultimately forced to buy them from their own pockets, they do not see any use in visiting the UHC. Even though this choice has a financial aspect, it also points to the institutional incapability of the UHC.

The respondent to this study has explained as follows:

> I visited Nachol Medical a month ago because of back pain. However, the medicine the UHC doctors prescribed was not available at that time. They told me to buy these medicines from an outside shop. The same had happened to me last year when I visited Nachol Medical for a fever and cold. One of my neighbors, who had recently visited the place for gastric problems, heard the same. They do not have the medicines in stock. Some medicines are always out of stock. It is very common now. The UHC authorities attempt to make extra money from selling medicines. As we are unable to pay for the medicines, they use this excuse of supply shortage. We would be surprised if someday they said they had all the medicines in stock. (EWL-5, in-depth interview on November 2, 2022)

As reported by the respondents to the study, most of the time the NUHC lacks the medicines that are prescribed to them by the doctors. This phenomenon plays an important role in limiting Santal women's preference for the UHC. This supply shortage issue can be interpreted as either the institutional incapacity of the whole public healthcare system of Bangladesh or the immoral intention of some of the healthcare authorities at the UHC to make some extra money, or both. Whatever the underlying reasons may be, this issue discourages the Santal women service recipients of the UHC from developing trust in the UHC services. The negative perception expressed by one of the respondents in the previous story is evidence of that. Similar results have been found by Islam et al. (2019) and Mannan (2013), as both of these two studies have identified a limited supply of medicine as a key barrier to healthcare accessibility.

Healing Hands in Short Supply: The Challenge of Health Provider Shortage

Another key institutional challenge hindering access to healthcare for Santal women is the shortage and absenteeism of doctors at the NUHC. Against the 16 sanctioned posts of junior consultants, the NUHC had only four posts filled in during the time of this investigation (DGHS, 2022). This lack of key health providers is a big challenge for the NUHC in providing health services. However, the NUHC cannot be blamed for this serious inadequacy for this shortage of doctors, as the doctors are appointed centrally. Even then, it cannot be avoided that the Santal women suffer greatly in accessing healthcare services due to doctor shortages. On top of the doctor shortage, those who are appointed to the NUHC are not very regular, as the respondents to the study expressed. Nachol Upazila is one of the backward places where doctors are very unlikely to come of their own volition. The respondents to this study have reported their dissatisfaction with the unavailability of doctors.

One of the Santal women interviewed for this study has responded:

I went to the NUHC a few months ago because of a lower belly ache. I had gone there early when the hospital opened. But no doctor was there. I had waited a while and then went to a private practitioner, as my pain was unbearable. The doctors of the NUHC usually come late and go early. Whenever we go to the hospital, we have to wait a long time to get to see a doctor. Many women from my village who had gone there had found the doctors absent. Some of the doctors rent houses in the town and spend much of their time there. Our area is not much developed, so they do not like to stay there, even sometimes ignoring their duty. (EWL-9, in-depth interview on November 2, 2022)

This story expresses the dissatisfaction of the healthcare recipients of the NUHC over the absenteeism of doctors. The number of health providers at NUHC is not satisfactory, as there are only five doctors appointed at the NUHC against 18 vacant posts (DGHS, 2022). This scenario is not unbelievable given the national average of doctors per patient ratio. At present, there are only 5.26 doctors for 10,000 patients in Bangladesh, which places the country in the second position from the bottom among South Asian countries (Bangladesh's health inclusivity, 2022). Those who are appointed are less likely to come to the facility regularly or on time. As Nachol is a peripheral area, doctors rent houses in the town and are irregular in their offices. This issue has demotivated the Santal women to visit the NUHC to seek healthcare. Adding to this, Reza et al. (2020) revealed in their study that a lack of medical resources and professionals, inadequate experience, and poor management have contributed to the uncontrolled transmission of the coronavirus in Bangladesh.

A number of other studies have identified the unavailability of doctors at public healthcare facilities as a major factor that demotivates people from accessing health services at rural public healthcare facilities. Khandakar (2014) has found that, among other factors, the availability of healthcare providers is a key determinant of patients' access to public healthcare. He further added that the lack of dedication to quality care by health professionals harms patients' safety. Another study by Rumi et al. (2021) supports this finding, as they suggest a poor doctor-patient ratio is an important determinant of patients' dissatisfaction with the UHCs. The issue of absenteeism among responsible health providers in the NUHC is evident, as it has been reported both by the respondents of the study and in the local and national dailies. The acting UH&FPO of NUHC has been irregular in her duties. Due to her unavailability in the office, the community clinics under NUHC have to fund their COVID-19 management measures all by themselves (Nachole Mathe nei, 2020). NUHC remained almost invisible with their inadequate COVID-19 management support for the root-level community clinics as well as the ethnic communities.

PAYING THE PRICE: SANTAL WOMEN'S FINANCIAL HURDLES AND DILEMMAS

The COVID-19 pandemic had the most significant setback to gender equality in history, regressively affecting women's economic and productive engagements. Any adverse effect on gender equality is undesirable because "what is good for gender equality is good for the economy and society" (Balagopal & Chacko, 2021). As economic barriers are one of the major hurdles to healthcare accessibility, the poorest segment of society is the largest user of public healthcare facilities. While the poor household has to spend 35% of their family income on an illness episode, it is only 5% for the rich segment. Thus, the costs incurred in accessing health services, including medicine, travel costs, pathological tests, and bribes, burden poor households heavily (Mannan, 2013). Traditionally, Santal households are reliant on lower-paying jobs. The COVID-19 virus has worsened the situation for Santals by negatively affecting their household incomes.[1] For most of the Santal women in this study, household income is the major source of healthcare financing. The income setbacks experienced during the pandemic have seriously affected the accessibility of healthcare for Santal women. The lack of institutional financial support in healthcare has made things worse for them.

The following section elaborately discusses the issue of financial challenges experienced by Santal women in accessing healthcare services.

Financial Accessibility to Healthcare During COVID-19

The outbreak of the COVID-19 pandemic has had a great negative impact on the income and financial status of people worldwide. Chattoraj et al. (2021), in their study on Rohingya refugees, found that, before the pandemic, girls worked as maids or in the local garment industry, while boys took on jobs like working at tea stalls and doing manual labor. However, the pandemic lockdowns significantly restricted their mobility, leading to economic difficulties, fear, and an uncertain future. The Santal women are no exception to this. The income and asset losses during the COVID-19 pandemic have made the Santal household, and hence Santal women,

---

[1] Household income of a Santal household is the total amount of money earned by all members of a single Santal household over a specific period (a year). It includes income from various sources, such as wages, government assistance, and other forms of earnings.

financially vulnerable. The reasons that play a direct role in this financial downturn are basically the movement restrictions and the increased healthcare costs of the health issues caused by the coronavirus. While Santal women earn their own income, they often have limited autonomy to spend it as they wish. Typically, they use their hard-earned money to cover family expenses and often need approval from their husbands or elders, especially for healthcare expenditures.

The following table illustrates how the pandemic has affected the financial situation of Santal women, Santal men, and non-ethnic women.

As is seen in Table 5.2, 26 (65%) of the Santal women have reported income loss during the coronavirus pandemic, whereas the numbers are 26 (65%) and 16 (40%) for the ethnic men and the non-ethnic women, respectively. Since they couldn't work in agriculture and/or as day laborers during the pandemic, they experienced significant income losses. The income loss of the 26 (65%) Santal men interviewed in this study was due to their inability to market their agricultural products. The non-ethnic women, on the contrary, had reported income loss as they were unable to go out because of the coronavirus lockdown. However, the male earning members of their family had gone out to earn, ignoring the COVID-19 lockdown. Twelve (30%) of the Santal women and (30%) of the non-ethnic women in the study have reported having sold their assets to deal with health issues.

A study by Molla and Chi (2017) suggests that most people in Bangladesh rely on out-of-pocket payments for their healthcare expenses. The Santals and other ethnic communities are no exception to this. Relying heavily on household income results in inequitable healthcare access, and the financial burden of healthcare affects the living standards of the people. The increase in income inequality caused by out-of-pocket payments is 89% (Molla & Chi, 2017). Affordability, along with availability and

Table 5.2 Changed financial status during COVID-19

Status	Santal women	Santal men	Non-ethnic women
Income loss	26 (65%)	26 (65%)	16 (40%)
Sold asset(s) for healthcare costs	12 (30%)	14 (35%)	12(30%)
Unchanged	2 (5%)	8 (20%)	12 (30%)
Total	40 (100%)	40 (100%)	40 (100%)

Source: Field research

accessibility, has been an important determinant of healthcare among the ethnic people of Bangladesh, including the Santals (Kumar Sarkar & Singha, 2019; Rahman et al., 2012). A field investigation suggests that the decreased financial status of Santal women has made them more vulnerable and weakened their position in their health-related decision-making. One of the primary effects of this can be seen in the decreased food intake and healthcare costs of Santal women. As reported by the respondents, the Santal women have become more aware of their healthcare needs after the coronavirus outbreak. This is one reason behind their increased healthcare costs in a time of financial uncertainty.

The following story better explains the financial hardships of Santal women in accessing healthcare during COVID-19:

> *I am 17 and I was carrying my first child during Corona. My mother-in-law got very sick back then, and as the female of the family, I had taken care of her. We thought she got corona, but the UHC doctors had said it was pneumonia. I usually earn money by working in the field with my husband. But I couldn't do it then. So, my whole family had to rely on my husband's very little income. It was quite hard for us to arrange food for all the family members. My husband was entitled to more or better food as the only earning member. The medicines of my mother-in-law had added to our monthly expenses. ... I didn't go through any treatment. Pregnancy is not a disease, and most of the Santal women do not go to the hospital for pregnancy care. But I have heard a nurse at the Nachol Medical say that if I had taken good food during the pregnancy, my child would have been healthy, and I wouldn't have to experience so many complications during childbirth.* (EWL-4, in-depth interview on November 2, 2022)

The interviews and Focus Group Discussions (FGDs) conducted in this study reveal that the economic condition of the Santals was already precarious before the COVID-19 pandemic. Unfortunately, the pandemic exacerbated their financial woes, putting their income at risk. This financial strain, coupled with their limited resources, often results in inadequate healthcare accessibility. The respondents in the study expressed genuine concern for the health of both Santal men and women. However, due to financial constraints, Santal women often find themselves sacrificing their healthcare needs, and their health concerns can go unaddressed, particularly in cases of extreme poverty. This situation serves as a poignant example of the difficult choices families face when resources are limited, making it challenging to prioritize the healthcare needs of multiple family members. In such circumstances, young Santal women may be dispropor-tionately overlooked, given their age and physical resilience.

Institutional Support in Healthcare Financing

As revealed in the previous discussion, financial affordability remains a prime factor in determining access to healthcare for Santal women. Financial factors directly and indirectly play a vital role in dominating the healthcare-seeking behavior of the respondents to the study. There are a series of costs involved in the process of receiving healthcare services. These fees include the doctor's fees, transportation costs, medicine costs, and the cost of pathological tests if required. The services at the UHC are less costly than those at other privately run healthcare facilities, but they are not entirely free. The costs incurred while accessing healthcare services are a key barrier for Santal women to access healthcare services, both public and private. In most Santal households, both men and women work as agricultural laborers to earn their livelihood. However, this monthly income is seldom enough to support their healthcare costs. In many instances, the Santal women have reported borrowing money from relatives and neighbors or taking loans from different sources to cover their health expenses.

Table 5.3 shows that the biggest source of healthcare finance for Santal women is their monthly household income. The majority of the Santal women interviewed in this study have a family income of 8000–12,000. With such little monthly income, it is hard to support a family let alone healthcare costs. Twelve (30%) of the Santal women have reported that frequently they had to rely on their relatives for loans in order to get healthcare during the COVID-19 outbreak and 10 (25%) of the Santal women said that they have taken loans from NGOs, cooperative societies,

Table 5.3 Santal women's sources of healthcare financing

Source of health finance	Santal women
Household income	18 (45%)
Loans from relatives	12 (30%)
Loans from other institutions	10 (25%)
Total	40 (100%)

Source: Field research

and other intuitions to support their healthcare. Interestingly, none of these institutions have any scheme for healthcare credit provision. These Santal women had to convince the authorities by expressing purposes other than health treatment in order to get the loan money. The respondents have reported that they wouldn't get the loan otherwise. The proportion of people taking credit from different institutions is nil for the Santal men and non-ethnic women.

The main source of money lenders among the respondents are NGOs. However, NGOs do not lend them money for treatment purposes. Some of the NGOs active in the locality have some programs for healthcare awareness, but they are not involved in giving healthcare credit and financing activities for ethnic people. NGOs issue loans for income-generating activities and not for treatment purposes. The Santal women thus take healthcare loans from the NGO reporting a different cause. This is a normal practice among the Santals as they have no other options available for providing healthcare credit. This single opportunity is also likely to vanish, as some NGOs like DASCOH foundation are strengthening their efforts to closely monitor if the money granted to the Santal women is used for the stated income-generating purpose. Some prominent NGOs like BRAC, Grameen Bank, Ashroy, and ASA are reported to not granting loans to people over 60 years of age because of the likelihood that they will die before repaying the loans.

Along with the NGOs and Christian missionary hospitals, there are a number of cooperative societies working to improve the life of Santal women. One of the most popular one is "Socio-economic development, savings and credit society for the Nachol thana aboriginal community" (*Nachol thana Adivasi jonogoshthir artho-samajik unnyan sonchoy o rindan somity*). This society for Santal people arranges skill development training for the Santal women and provides credit for income-generating activities. However, they do not provide any healthcare loans to the Santals. The healthcare needs especially of the Santal women are largely overlooked by their own community and organization as it was believed by the authorities of this society that Santals do not usually get sick and so health credit system and health services are not that important for the Santals, even for women who need healthcare support for menstruation and menopause-related health issues, malnutrition, anemia, and pregnancy-related treatment even if they are less prone to contract other illnesses.

One respondent of this study has expressed

*I am too old to work in the agricultural field along with my nephew and his wife, with whom I stay. I don't have kids of my own. Although I am old and incapable of working, I do not get any allowance from the government. Most of the **cards** (social safety net allowance cards) are given to the people close to the local politicians, even to those who have big houses and plenty of money. Families in our village starve two-three days in a row during **Ashwin maas** (a month in Bengali calendar) due to lack of work and food. NGOs however will not grant me loans as I am old and likely to die without repaying their loan with interest. NGOs push us to take loans and then squeeze us for the interest money. One of my brothers was forced to take a loan of 12,000 BDT from an NGO and had to repay an interest of 9000 BDT. The NGO's attitude is like **khudi diye murgi dhora** (spreading rice as a trap to catch chickens). Once you are in, you are in huge debt in no time. NGOs are only concerned with their own profit and not with the welfare of our people. They allow loans for income-generating activities but not for healthcare. One of my nieces who needed loans for her T.B. treatment thus made an excuse of opening a shop and finally get the credit to treat her illness.* (EWH 18, in-depth interview on October 20, 2022)

This story reveals that proper healthcare is a luxury to the Santal women living in acute poverty. On top of that, they have little or no institutional support to finance their health costs. The cheap health services provided by the UHC are hard for them to access, often due to their disadvantaged social identity and sometimes because of the overall expenses they need to bear in accessing the services. Even though the healthcare costs incurred at the UHC are significantly cheap, the hidden costs involved in the health seeking from the UHC (transportation cost, for example) make it too much for the Santal women to bear. Santals as a community in general are poor. Affordability to healthcare is thus a big challenge for them. In order to get proper treatment, they often have to take loans from their relatives and other institutions like the NGOs. However, the NGOs working in the area have no such scheme for granting healthcare loans to the Santals. Borrowed money from relatives is not always adequate to support their health costs as their relatives are not richer than themselves. Thus, unaffordability remains a prime cause in Santal women's access to healthcare.

Language and Communication Barrier

Language barriers can hinder effective communication between patients and healthcare providers, leading to misunderstandings and potentially compromising the quality of care. Patients who face language barriers may be less likely to seek medical help, leading to delayed or inadequate treatment. Additionally, healthcare providers may struggle to accurately assess patients' symptoms and medical history, impacting diagnosis and treatment decisions. Olani et al. (2023) suggest that patients experience preventable medical errors, low adherence to treatment, reduced health-seeking behavior, increased treatment costs, longer hospital stays, weakened therapeutic relationships, social desirability bias, lower confidence, and dissatisfaction with healthcare. For healthcare providers, language barriers hinder their ability to gather patient history, make diagnoses, provide treatment, and increase their workload. Another study by Al Shamsi et al. (2020) suggests that language barriers in healthcare contribute to miscommunication between medical professionals and patients, resulting in reduced satisfaction and compromised healthcare quality and patient safety.

During the COVID-19 pandemic, Santal women faced significant healthcare access challenges rooted in language and cultural barriers. These obstacles were deeply intertwined with the unique cultural context of the Santal community, creating difficulties in engaging with healthcare services. Language barriers were a prominent issue among these challenges. Santal women often had limited proficiency in Bengali, the dominant language in healthcare settings. This language gap made it challenging for them to effectively communicate their symptoms and understand medical guidance. This communication barrier could lead to misunderstandings and potentially compromise the quality of care they received. Cultural traditions also played a substantial role. Santal women felt more comfortable seeking healthcare from traditional healers who were fluent in Santali and well-versed in their cultural practices. These indigenous health practitioners are aligned with Santal cultural norms and beliefs, making them a preferred choice for healthcare. This preference provided an alternative to formal healthcare, as traditional healers offered services in Santali and respected Santal cultural traditions. However, Lima et al. (2021) suggest that marginalized communities did not choose to seek medical assistance from unqualified practitioners or pharmacies; rather, they were forced to do so due to the pre-existing financial marginalization exaggerated by the COVID-19 outbreak.

One of the respondents of the study has asserted:

When I got sick during the pandemic, I had trouble talking to doctors because they mostly spoke Bengali, a language I wasn't very good at. It made it hard for me to explain what was wrong, and I was worried they might not understand me correctly. So, I decided to visit a traditional healer who spoke my native Santali language. When I went to the traditional healer's place, I immediately felt more comfortable. They listened carefully while I talked about how I was feeling in Santali, and I could see in their eyes that they understood. They gave me the right treatment for our culture, and I trusted them completely. My experience made me realize how important it is for healthcare to understand different languages and cultures so that everyone can get the care they need. (EWH-3, in-depth interview on 02 November 2022)

Another respondent has asserted:

You see, I primarily spoke Santali, a language deeply rooted in our Santal culture. But at the health complex, they primarily communicated in Bengali. The thought of trying to explain my symptoms and concerns in a language I wasn't comfortable with was terrifying. I feared that I wouldn't be able to accurately convey my condition's seriousness. It felt like an insurmountable barrier, and I couldn't help but think about when I struggled to understand the healthcare workers during previous visits. The fear of misunderstanding and the frustration of not being able to express myself properly were overwhelming. I was torn between seeking medical help for my deteriorating health and the language challenge that awaited me at the health complex. The uncertainty demotivated me. (EWL-3, in-depth interview on 02 November 2022)

The discussion above suggests that Santal women experience language barriers in seeking healthcare. This cannot be said for Santal women uniquely because studies conducted in other countries such as Ethiopia and Oman also suggest similar findings. In addition to linguistic differences, supportive communication by the health providers also plays a key role in determining the healthcare behavior of the patients. In this context, Zakaria et al. (2021) have revealed that Bengali patients generally received more supportive communication behaviors from Bengali doctors compared to ethnic minority patients in Bangladesh. These behaviors included cheerful greetings, encouraging patients to express health problems, active listening, responding to questions and concerns, explaining medical procedures and medications, discussing treatment options, involving patients in decisions, and spending adequate time with them.

Challenges in Accessing Telemedicine Service

Telemedicine services have emerged as a critical lifeline in healthcare access during the COVID-19 pandemic (Chowdhury et al., 2020; Khan et al., 2021). This innovative approach to healthcare delivery has played a pivotal role in ensuring that patients continue to receive essential medical care while adhering to social distancing guidelines and reducing the risk of viral transmission. One of the most significant advantages of telemedicine is its ability to bridge the physical gap between patients and healthcare providers, enabling timely consultations and medical advice without the need for in-person visits to hospitals or clinics (Khan et al., 2021). In addition, telemedicine has also played a significant role in rural and underserved areas where healthcare access was already limited before the pandemic. By eliminating the need for long travel distances and enabling consultations from the comfort of one's home, telemedicine has helped mitigate healthcare disparities and reach patients who previously faced barriers to receiving medical care.

During the pandemic, telemedicine has proven its importance in maintaining continuity of care for individuals with chronic conditions (Khan et al., 2021). Patients with conditions like diabetes, hypertension, and heart disease can receive regular check-ups, medication adjustments, and disease management guidance through virtual consultations. This not only helps in preventing disease exacerbation but also reduces the burden on overwhelmed healthcare facilities that need to prioritize COVID-19 cases. Furthermore, patients with mild symptoms or those seeking guidance on testing and quarantine measures can consult healthcare professionals remotely, reducing unnecessary visits to healthcare facilities and curbing the potential spread of the virus.

Santal women in Nachol Upazila, Bangladesh, faced a multitude of barriers when seeking access to telemedicine services during the COVID-19 pandemic. These barriers encompassed technological limitations, cultural considerations, language disparities, and challenges related to health literacy and gender norms. Many Santal women lacked access to the necessary digital tools, such as smartphones or computers with internet connectivity, which are fundamental for engaging in telemedicine consultations. This digital divide is intensifying the difficulty Santal women face in participating in remote healthcare services. Language presented another significant hurdle. Moreover, telemedicine services in NUHC predominantly operate in the Bengali language, which, in most cases, is not the primary language for Santal women. Language barriers likely obstruct effective communication of their health concerns and comprehension of medical advice during telehealth consultations. Furthermore, geographical constraints compounded the issue. Nachol Upazila, like many rural areas, grappled with geographical remoteness and inadequate infrastructure, including unreliable internet access. As a result, it has been difficult for village dwellers to use mobile phones and the Internet to seek healthcare.

The following table illustrates the potential reasons identified by the study respondents behind their inability to access telemedicine services during the COVID-19 pandemic (Table 5.4).

The field investigation of this study has revealed that the majority of the Santal women (18, 45%) interviewed in this study believed a lack of digital literacy and language barriers to be the major reasons behind their inability to access telemedicine services during the pandemic. Ten (25%) others thought that lack of technology and connectivity was the main problem, and the rest 12 (30%) Santal women thought that financial limitation was their key constraining factor for not being able to access telemedicine services during the pandemic outbreak. The responses of Santal men are almost similar to those of Santal women. They too identify digital literacy and language barriers as the key constraints on accessing telehealth services amid the COVID-19 outbreak. Non-ethnic women, on the contrary, have identified a lack of technology and connectivity as the major issue behind their inaccessibility.

The NUHC has a telemedicine service in its eyecare center, where patients can take expert suggestions (where required) at a minimum expense. The NUHC health providers manage this service delivery under

Table 5.4 Factors limiting Santal women's access to telemedicine service

Key barriers to accessing telemedicine service	Santal women (n = 40)	Santal men (n = 40)	Non-ethnic women (n = 40)
Lack of technology and connectivity	10 (25%)	7 (17.5%)	24 (60%)
Digital literacy and language barriers	18 (45%)	21 (52.5%)	6 (15%)
Financial constraints	12 (30%)	12 (30%)	10 (25%)
Total	40 (100%)	40 (100%)	40 (100%)

Source: Field investigation

their supervision and guidance. However, the KII of this study with one of the health providers at the NUHC has revealed that the non-ethnic population of Nachol are the main service seekers at the telemedicine center where telemedicine service is offered. The Santal population is quite hesitant to accept the service.

She reported:

> *Santals, especially Santal women, rarely come to our hospital to access the telemedicine services we offer. Maybe it's because of their fear of technology. We have run several campaigns to encourage them to take telemedicine services among others, but these efforts were not very fruitful. They have very little or no knowledge of technology, as a result, they are fearful to use it.* (EWH-2, in-depth interview on October 20, 2022)

When asked about their access to telemedicine services during the COVID-19 lockdown, Santal women responded as follows:

> *During the pandemic, our family had only one smartphone, but my teenage son kept it for his entertainment. I fell sick, hoping to consult a doctor through telehealth, but he wouldn't share the phone. I felt helpless, unable to access healthcare, and feared it might be COVID-19. Eventually, I borrowed a neighbor's phone to consult a doctor, who diagnosed me with a severe flu. Having another phone could help me avoid feeling hopeless and anxious in the troubling situation of Corona.* (EWL-6, in-depth interview on 02 November 2022)

Another woman reported:

> *During the COVID-19 pandemic, I found myself facing significant challenges due to our family's lack of a smartphone. This seemingly small device had become a lifeline for us, providing access to updated COVID-19 information and crucial telehealth services. But with no smartphone in our household, I was cut off from the latest news and guidelines. The ever-changing situation left me feeling anxious and isolated. Lockdown measures were in place, restricting our movements and preventing us from visiting healthcare facilities in person. This made telehealth services our best option for seeking medical advice and assistance. However, without the necessary technology, this option remained out of reach.* (EWH-7, in-depth interview on October 20, 2022)

The qualitative evidence presented above expresses that Santal women had very little access to technology, a low level of digital literacy, and a fear of using technology, which restricted them from accessing telemedicine services during the coronavirus outbreak. The field investigation of the present study could record the Santal women's view on factors they perceive as most important in limiting their telemedicine access. However, since the Santal community could rarely use telemedicine services during the COVID-19 outbreak, it was not possible to measure or compare their level and extent of telemedicine accessibility. Rahman et al. (2022) in their study on gender disparity in telehealth usage in Bangladesh during COVID-19 have found that male patients had a higher reliance on telehealth compared to females. They believe that differences in education levels and technical skills contribute to gender disparities in accessing telehealth services. Lack of technical literacy, coupled with limited awareness of online platforms, contributes to the gender gap in accessing telehealth services, as women, especially from older age groups, may face more significant challenges in utilizing digital healthcare solutions. Adding to the challenges reported by the Santal women respondents of this study, Rahman et al. (2020) have found that low trustworthiness, difficulties accessing emergency diagnostic services, anxiety about the complexity and observability of telemedicine, network, and power supply issues, and financial challenges are the key constraints in accessing telemedicine services during the COVID-19 pandemic in Bangladesh.

CONCLUSION

This chapter briefly explains the institutional, linguistic, and technological challenges experienced by Santal women in accessing healthcare services. Institutional challenges that have hindered Santal women's healthcare accessibility during the COVID-19 outbreak include the failure of NUHC health providers to identify the poor segment of the community, absenteeism and inadequate number of health providers, and a shortage of medicines at the NUHC. Santal women are by and large poor. On top of that, there is a serious lack of financial support for healthcare from NGOs and non-profit organizations. Thus, high out-of-pocket payment occurs in accessing healthcare that either discourages the Santal women from accessing healthcare services or encourages them to ignore their healthcare needs. The health behavior of the Santal women dominated by the poor level of health literacy, lack of technical know-how in accessing telemedicine services, and the discriminatory treatment by the NUHC health providers limited the healthcare accessibility of the poor Santal women during the coronavirus pandemic.

REFERENCES

Al Shamsi, H., Almutairi, A. G., Al Mashrafi, S., & Al Kalbani, T. (2020). Implications of language barriers for healthcare: A systematic review. *Oman Medical Journal, 35*(2), e122.

Balagopal, B., & Chacko, J. P. (2021). The pandemic crisis and economic engagement of women: A historical enquiry on implications of catastrophes on female economic participation. In I. George & M. Kuruvilla (Eds.), *Gendered experiences of COVID-19 in India.* Palgrave Macmillan. https://doi.org/10.1007/978-3-030-85335-8_2

Bangladesh's health inclusivity. (2022, October 16). *The Financial Express.* Retrieved December 20, 2023, from https://thefinancialexpress.com.bd/editorial/bangladeshs-health-inclusivity-16659309988

Biswas, R. K., Huq, S., Afiaz, A., & Khan, H. T. A. (2020). A systematic assessment on COVID-19 preparedness and transition strategy in Bangladesh. *Journal of Evaluation in Clinical Practice, 26*(6), 1599–1611. https://doi.org/10.1111/jep.13467

Chattoraj, D., Ullah, A. A. K. M., & Hossain, M. A. (2021). The COVID-19 pandemic and the travails of Rohingya Refugees in the largest Bangladeshi Refugee camp. In B. Doucet, R. van Melik, & P. Filion (Eds.), *Global reflections on COVID-19 and cities: Urban inequalities in the age of pandemic.* Bristol University Policy Press.

Chowdhury, S. R., Sunna, T. C., & Ahmed, S. (2020). Telemedicine is an important aspect of healthcare services amid COVID-19 outbreak: Its barriers in Bangladesh and strategies to overcome. *The International Journal of Health Planning and Management, 36*(1), 4–12. https://doi.org/10.1002/hpm.3064

DGHS. (2022). Nachol Upazila Health Complex HRM status. Retrieved October 16, 2022, from http://facilityregistry.dghs.gov.bd/hrm_status.php?org_code=100011688

Islam, M. Z., Zaman, F., Farjana, S., & Khanam, S. (2019). Accessibility to health care services of Upazila Health Complex: Experience of rural people. *Journal of Preventive and Social Medicine, 38*(2), 30–37.

Islam, S., Islam, R., Mannan, F., Rahman, S., & Islam, T. (2020). COVID-19 pandemic: An analysis of the healthcare, social and economic challenges in Bangladesh. *Progress in Disaster Science, 8*, 100135. https://doi.org/10.1016/j.pdisas.2020.100135

Khan, M. M., Rahman, S. M. T., & Anjum Islam, S. T. (2021). The use of telemedicine in Bangladesh during COVID-19 pandemic. *E-Health Telecommunication Systems and Networks, 10*(1). https://doi.org/10.4236/etsn.2021.101001

Khandakar, M. S. A. (2014). Rural health care system and patients' satisfaction towards medical care in Bangladesh: An empirical study. *Journal of Business Studies, 35*(2).

Kumar Sarkar, A., & Singha, S. (2019). Factors influencing health of the Santals: A study of selected villages of Birbhum. *The International Journal of Community and Social Development, 1*(1), 58–74.

Lima, T. R., Ela, M. Z., Khan, L., Shovo, T. E. A., Hossain, M. T., Jahan, N., Rahman, K. S., Ahsan, M. N., & Islam, M. N. (2021). Livelihood and health vulnerabilities of forest resource-dependent communities amidst the COVID-19 pandemic in southwestern regions of Bangladesh. In A. L. Ramanathan, C. Sabarathinam, F. Arriola, M. V. Prasanna, P. Kumar, & M. P. Jonathan (Eds.), *Environmental resilience and transformation in times of COVID-19* (pp. 343–356). Elsevier. https://doi.org/10.1016/B978-0-323-85512-9.00027-9

Mannan, M. A. (2013). Access to public health facilities in Bangladesh: A study on facility utilisation and burden of treatment. *The Bangladesh Development Studies, 36*(4).

Molla, A. A., & Chi, C. (2017). Who pays for healthcare in Bangladesh? An analysis of progressivity in health systems financing. *International Journal for Equity in Health, 16*(1), 1–10.

Nachole Mathe nei Upazila Shashtho o Poribar Porikolpona kormokorta Sultana Papia. (2020, March 27). *The Daily Inqilab.* https://m.dailyinqilab.com/article/278691/

Olani, A. B., Olani, A. B., Muleta, T. B., Rikitu, D. H., & Disassa, K. G. (2023). Impacts of language barriers on healthcare access and quality among Afaan Oromoo-speaking patients in Addis Ababa, Ethiopia. *BMC Health Services Research, 23.* https://doi.org/10.1186/s12913-023-09036-z

Rahman, Q. M., Rahman, M. E., Aziz, R., Pranta, M. U. R., Zubayer, A. A., Islam, M. B., Bhuiyan, M. R. A. M., Khan, K. A., Chowdhury, A. U., & Hosain, L. (2020). Perceptions and barriers regarding telemedicine services among Bangladeshi young adults in the COVID-19 pandemic: A qualitative exploration. *Asian Journal of Health Sciences, 6*(2). https://doi.org/10.15419/ajhs.v6i2.477

Rahman, S., Amit, S., & Al Kafy, A. A. (2022). Gender disparity in telehealth usage in Bangladesh during COVID-19. *SSM—Mental Health, 2,* 100054. https://doi.org/10.1016/j.ssmmh.2021.100054

Rahman, S. A., Tara Kielmann, B. M. P., & Normand, C. (2012). Healthcare-seeking behaviour among the tribal people of Bangladesh: Can the current health system really meet their needs? *Journal of Health, Population, and Nutrition, 30*(3), 353.

Reza, H. M., Sultana, F., & Khan, I. O. (2020). Disruption of healthcare amid COVID-19 pandemic in Bangladesh. *The Open Public Health Journal, 13,* 438–440. https://doi.org/10.2174/1874944502013010438

Rumi, M. H., Makhdum, N., Rashid, M. H., & Muyeed, A. (2021). Patients' satisfaction on the service quality of Upazila Health Complex in Bangladesh. *Journal of Patient Experience, 8.*

Zakaria, M., Karim, R., Rahman, M., Cheng, F., & Xu, J. (2021). Disparity in physician-patient communication by ethnicity: Evidence from Bangladesh. *International Journal for Equity in Health, 20*(1). https://doi.org/10.1186/s12939-021-01405-6

Unlocking New Perspectives: Lessons and Future Avenues

Abstract This chapter highlights the summary of the key findings of the study. It discusses how the current research has addressed the theoretical and evidence gaps in the current scholarships of access to health and ensured the inclusion of Santal women's healthcare access in the academic discourse. This chapter finally reveals the way to shape government and healthcare policies to promote Santal women's accessibility to healthcare and how future research could contribute to this area.

Keywords Key findings • Policy suggestions • Future research

The right to health is recognized by all states in the world (WHO, 2022). The issues of gender equality, non-discrimination, and accessibility of health services, goods, and facilities are recognized in all major global health-related treaties. However, access to healthcare for ethnic women in Bangladesh remains a complex and multifaceted challenge within the realm of public health. The prevailing policies governing healthcare provision in Bangladesh often encounter numerous perplexities when intersecting with the dimensions of ethnic identity. The Santal community, an ethnic minority in the country, grapples with inherent socio-cultural barriers that impede their access to essential healthcare services (Macdonald,

© The Author(s), under exclusive license to Springer Nature Switzerland AG 2023
F. Nawaz, AN Bushra, *Santal Women and the Health Care Regime*,
https://doi.org/10.1007/978-3-031-48872-6_6

2021). This conundrum demands a nuanced examination of the intricacies involved, where factors such as linguistic diversity, cultural norms, and
geographic disparities intertwine. Despite significant strides in healthcare
policies and initiatives, the full realization of the right to health for ethnic
women remains a formidable task.

This chapter employs a two-part structure to present its content. The
first part focuses on highlighting significant findings and their academic
contributions to the existing body of knowledge. The second part offers
informed speculations regarding healthcare policies as well as potential
directions for future research endeavors. It delves into areas concerning
access to services among ethnic minorities and the crucial pursuit of equitable healthcare access. The study informs us that socio-economic status
and the complex interplay of social identity play a pivotal role in shaping
healthcare behavior and the ability to access healthcare services for
Santal women.

The empirical findings derived from this investigation have made a substantial and noteworthy contribution to the existing corpus of knowledge.
This research, situated at the juncture of theoretical and practical realms,
has bestowed an invaluable addition to the literature concerning the
domains of public health, healthcare accessibility, and healthcare service.
Moreover, it has imparted novel insights into the discourse of gender and
social justice by meticulously examining the experiential narratives of
diverse gender and ethnic cohorts. Equally salient is the methodological
prowess exhibited in this study. Henceforth, the preponderance of inqui-
ries scrutinizing the healthcare access of ethnic women has leaned heavily
toward quantitative research paradigms, characterized by the deployment
of surveys and questionnaires as data-gathering instruments. On the other
hand, qualitative investigations delving into ethnic communities' healthcare encounters have predominantly relied upon secondary sources. These
pre-existing studies, to a large extent, have identified varying factors influencing healthcare accessibility while eschewing the pursuit of an in-depth
comprehension of ethnic women's access, which this current research ear-
nestly endeavors to achieve.

While the ideal of universal healthcare for all women remains sanguine,
practicality demonstrates that merely a paltry cohort of mainstream women
truly possess the empowered gateway to public healthcare services.
Observations from the empirical realm underscore that numerous Santal
women respondents' roles in familial healthcare decision-making are tenu-
ous, rendering them reticent toward acknowledging their healthcare

exigencies. The salient findings emanating from the study are thus encapsulated as follows:

1. The findings of this book point out a concerning trend among Santal women, highlighting that a higher percentage of them opted for public healthcare facilities (UHC) once or twice as compared to private ones. However, the situation changes when considering multiple visits, with more Santal women revisiting private healthcare facilities. This shift suggests growing trust in private healthcare due to positive experiences. This study also reveals pronounced disparities in healthcare seeking across Santal women, Santal men, and non-ethnic women. Non-ethnic women display a greater inclination toward private healthcare, whereas Santal men have better access to private facilities than Santal women. Moreover, existing unequal treatment, nepotism, and favoritism within public healthcare institutions are especially affecting Santal women. It points out that Santal women are less likely to protest against institutional irregularities, partly due to their poor self-image and the normalization of discrimination.

2. Lower levels of education among Santal women make them susceptible to misinformation and misconceptions about the pandemic. With only 9% having literacy and 2% completing secondary education, illiteracy is prevalent among minority ethnic groups like the Santals. This educational disparity contributes to their vulnerability to fake news and rumors about COVID-19. In addition to this, high levels of trust and stigma play significant roles in influencing the information-seeking behaviors and attitudes of Santal women toward healthcare systems. The stigma associated with COVID-19 in their community has led some Santal women to hide their symptoms, fearing discrimination. Trust in government vaccination campaigns and NGOs has played a crucial role in overcoming fear and misinformation. Some Santal women expressed fear and mistrust related to COVID-19 stigma, while others emphasized their reliance on community health workers and NGO professionals for accurate information and guidance.

3. Some positive behaviors have pervaded the Santal community during the COVID-19 pandemic. Safe sanitary practices and cleanliness are two of them. This positive change has been possible with the support of a number of NGOs and government entities to

promote public health awareness through information dissemination and providing tools and kits needed for healthy sanitary practices. However, these supports are momentary measures. No long-term plans or programs have been made to preserve this positive change in attitude and behavior among the Santal women. The NGOs and cooperative societies active in the area have been reported not to issue healthcare loans, which is an acutely felt need of the Santal women.

4. Despite their generally negative perception of Nachol Upazila Health Complex (NUHC) services, Santal women have demonstrated high participation rates in the COVID-19 vaccination program. This is attributed to the commendable role played by NUHC in managing the COVID-19 crisis, with support from local voluntary organizations and NGOs. The NUHC, along with these community actors, actively raised awareness, disseminated information, and conducted vaccination campaigns, leading to successful vaccination coverage among Santal women. The data in Table 4.5 illustrates that Santal women's vaccination rates are slightly higher than those of non-ethnic women, due to the extensive awareness-building efforts carried out in Santal villages. The respondents in the study express their gratitude for the collective efforts of various stakeholders, including NGOs, local health workers, and community volunteers, in combating the pandemic.

5. During the COVID-19 pandemic, Santal women faced significant healthcare access challenges due to language and cultural barriers. Many of them had limited proficiency in Bengali, the dominant language in healthcare settings, which made it difficult for them to communicate their symptoms and understand medical advice. Cultural preferences led some Santal women to seek care from traditional healers who spoke Santali and understood their cultural practices. However, this reliance on traditional healers also stemmed from financial constraints, as marginalized communities like the Santal struggled to access formal healthcare due to financial limitations exacerbated by the pandemic. Access to telemedicine services during the pandemic posed additional challenges for Santal women, including a lack of digital tools and digital literacy. These barriers highlight the need for targeted interventions to address language, cultural, and technological issues and ensure

equitable healthcare access for marginalized communities, particularly women.

6. Some institutional inefficiency is also important to address in order to promote the healthcare accessibility of the Santal women. Insufficient doctors and a shortage of medicines are found to be the major institutional barriers behind the Santal women's poor access to healthcare. The discriminatory behavior of the health providers of the NUHC has been reported by 18 (45%) Santal women as a demotivating factor behind their health-seeking. Previous encounters with the health providers of the NUHC have discouraged the Santal women from seeking healthcare from the NUHC, and the financial condition of the Santals does not permit them to choose private hospitals as a healthcare destination. Thus, they prefer to ignore their healthcare needs on many occasions or rely on traditional health providers. Six (15%) of the respondents of the study have reported that the doctors are often absent and they have to wait long hours to meet the doctors. And 10 (25%) of them have reported the unavailability of medicines as their prime cause for not seeking healthcare from the NUHC. The efforts of NUHC to promote health awareness and ensure the inclusivity of Santal women in healthcare have been inefficient due to their focus on areas where the Santal people are in a better position financially, ignoring the poor segment of the community.

7. Our investigation highlights a significant relationship between health service utilization and individuals' personal health practices, health behaviors, and recognition of healthcare needs. Consistent with Anderson's model, our study also supports the importance of healthcare outcomes in influencing health behavior and healthcare needs. Moreover, our research provides additional evidence for the model's feedback loop, which intricately connects health outcomes, health behavior, and population characteristics. Notably, our findings reveal how negative experiences at the Nachol Upazila Health Complex (NUHC) have discouraged Santal women from returning to seek health services there, while private healthcare facilities have had the opposite effect. Respondents' healthcare needs were influenced by their previous encounters and available resources, with the cost of private healthcare and discriminatory treatment and inefficiency at the NUHC shaping their perceptions.

8. The present study explores the intersectional model, which suggests that individuals possess intricate and multifaceted identities shaped by interconnected factors. These identities can lead to experiences of discrimination or privilege within society. In the context of healthcare access, the study specifically examines the experiences of Santal women. The intersection of gender and ethnicity compounds the discrimination faced by Santal women, both within their own community and when interacting with healthcare facilities. Surprisingly, health providers tend to display more discriminatory behaviors toward Santal women compared to Santal men, resulting in a gender advantage for the latter. Interestingly, women from non-ethnic backgrounds who share a similar socioeconomic status with Santal women report encountering fewer discriminatory incidents with health providers, as found in the field investigation of this study.

9. By offering empirical evidence derived from firsthand field data through an in-depth qualitative approach, this study stands out from previous research on healthcare accessibility for the impoverished. It fills methodological and conceptual gaps prevalent in the literature and contributes significantly to existing theories. This novel qualitative study sheds light on the unequal access to healthcare services experienced by ethnic women in Bangladesh, a topic that has been underexplored in the existing literature. Moreover, the review of the literature highlights the scarcity of studies exclusively focusing on the healthcare needs of ethnic women and the absence of research adopting an intersectional framework to examine the healthcare accessibility of disadvantaged rural women in Bangladesh. As a result, this study introduces a fresh perspective and methodology, making a substantial and noteworthy addition to the existing body of knowledge.

10. The field investigation identifies manageable barriers to healthcare accessibility, requiring adequate policy measures and proper implementation for resolution. Recommendations are made to enhance healthcare access for Santal women. Ambiguities in some government health policies regarding de facto inequality in the healthcare system necessitate clearer explanations to ensure equality and inclusivity. Improving healthcare accessibility for ethnic women in Bangladesh involves steps such as emphasizing inclusive healthcare in government documents and policies, addressing the healthcare

needs of ethnic communities living on the mainland, introducing healthcare loans and insurance facilities, and disseminating health information effectively considering the education level of the target population. Increasing healthcare budget allocation, promoting cooperation between government and non-government actors, and addressing discriminatory practices by healthcare providers are also vital for efficient health management and public healthcare service delivery. Introducing reforms to enhance accountability and prevent mismanagement of public funds further contributes to improved healthcare provision.

Enriching Academic Discourse

The findings of this study have significantly contributed to the existing body of knowledge. This research is of both theoretical and practical significance and adds to the existing literature pertaining to public health, healthcare accessibility, and healthcare service. It has also added to gender and social justice literature by discussing the experiences of different gender and ethnic groups. In addition, the thesis also has methodological value. So far, the majority of research exploring the access to healthcare of ethnic women in Bangladesh has used quantitative research methods; surveys and questionnaires have been applied as data collection tools (Khandakar, 2014; Ame et al., 2021; Islam & Odland, 2011; Ali et al., 2016). Qualitative studies on ethnic people's healthcare are mostly based on ethnic communities in CHT (Akter et al., 2020). These literatures by and large have identified different factors of healthcare accessibility but didn't try to gain an in-depth understanding of ethnic women's access, which this research study has aimed to do. The qualitative research methods and data collection tools used have enabled this study to achieve a detailed and in-depth understanding of the problem concerned.

Chapter 3 of this book deliberates upon the limitations inherent in prevailing theoretical models of healthcare accessibility and has identified gaps within the extant literature. The empirical outcomes of the present study both align with and diverge from certain established theories and models. Levesque's Conceptual Framework of Access to Health, for instance, contends that an individual's capacity to seek healthcare is determined by personal and social values, cultural influences, and gender dynamics (Levesque et al., 2013). Nonetheless, this investigation reveals that the influence of gender and cultural identity extends beyond the realm of mere accessibility, occasionally permeating the stages of health-care attainment and utilization. The study underscores that ethnic women confront challenges of restricted mobility and affordability in terms of transportation, impacting their ability to access healthcare services. Furthermore, the study underscores that social norms and ethnicity act as constraints on the mobility of Santal women, consequently diminishing their healthcare access, a facet not encompassed within Levesque's frame-work. Moreover, upon reaching healthcare facilities, instances arise where these women are unable to effectively utilize the available healthcare ser-vices due to illiteracy and prejudicial treatment meted out by healthcare providers, a consequence of their marginalized societal status. Consequently, it is evident that factors of gender and other components of social identity exert significant influence throughout all stages of this access model.

Levesque's model does not comprehensively elucidate the nuanced interplay of genetic, ethnic, and political variables as pivotal determinants and influencers of healthcare requirements within populations. Furthermore, the model's absence of a feedback mechanism impedes the establishment of a cohesive linkage between health outcomes, healthcare needs, and the populace's perception thereof. The present study discerns that an individual's health-seeking behavior is significantly shaped by their prior interactions with healthcare providers and the quality of services encountered. This phenomenon is particularly evident in the preference of Santal women for private healthcare alternatives over public facilities, pre-dominantly rooted in unsatisfactory past encounters. Consequently, it becomes evident that a feedback loop is integral to individuals' healthcare access, a facet not encompassed within Levesque's model. This research corroborates the pivotal role of historical experiences or feedback mecha-nisms within the context of perceiving healthcare needs, fostering the desire for care, and shaping the subsequent healthcare-seeking trajectory within the framework of Levesque's model.

One of the shortcomings of Andersen's healthcare utilization model is this model fails to address cases in which people's healthcare need is real-ized and healthcare services are available but they still can't attain health-care services (Andersen, 1995). The behavior of health providers is also absent from this model. It was found in this study that, although the healthcare institutions are within the reach of the people and there is a complete healthcare system in Bangladesh, they are not always efficient in addressing the patient's needs. This study suggests that the inefficiencies of a healthcare system often determine the healthcare-seeking of a community. However, this issue is not discussed in this model. As per the current study, institutional inefficiencies determining health-seeking behavior and healthcare accessibility are inadequate number of health providers and shortage of medicines. Other aspects of this model are in conformity with the findings of the study.

This book suggests that health service utilization is closely related to personal health practices, health behaviors, and healthcare and needs recognition. Anderson's model depicts the same. Also, the role of healthcare outcomes in determining healthcare needs and health behavior is another aspect of this model that supports the findings of the present study. The role of the feedback loop in this model is to connect health outcomes with health behavior and population characteristics. The current study is in conformity with this aspect as well. In the present study, it was found that poor experience at the NUHC has discouraged Santal women from going back to the Upazila Health Complex (UHC) for health, and the opposite has happened in the case of private healthcare facilities. In the study, respondents perceived their healthcare needs based on their prior experiences and resources. Their healthcare needs are shaped by the unaffordability of private healthcare, discriminatory treatment, and inefficient services at the NUHC. Thus, the findings of the present study support the feedback loop as well.

The intersectional model assumes that human beings are exposed to multiple identity factors that intersect and/or overlap to produce a more complex identity, based on which they are either discriminated against or privileged in a socio-political setting. The findings of this study are very much in conformity with intersectionality theory. Santal women are discriminated against in their access to healthcare based on their intersecting identities of gender and ethnicity. Santal women are disadvantaged in both their community and the healthcare facilities, where the health providers have shown discriminatory treatment toward Santal women more often than in the case of Santal men. Santal men enjoy a comparative gender advantage over Santal women in healthcare facilities. On the other hand, poor non-ethnic women of similar socio-economic backgrounds as the Santal women of the study have reported experiencing little discriminatory comments from the health providers.

The Santal community, characterized by a patriarchal social structure, sees both male and female members actively participating in agricultural labor. However, the COVID-19 pandemic exposed how this social structure perpetuates inequalities and hinders the equitable distribution of benefits within the community. While both genders contribute to agricultural work, the pandemic exacerbated the pre-existing vulnerabilities and disparities faced by Santal women. They continued to engage in strenuous agricultural activities during the crisis, often alongside their male counterparts, but their labor did not translate into commensurate benefits or recognition within the household or the community. The intersectional perspective reveals that Santal women faced a unique set of challenges during the pandemic, including language and cultural barriers to accessing healthcare services, limited digital literacy, and the burden of domestic responsibilities. These intersecting factors compounded the adverse effects of the pandemic, underscoring the urgent need for gender-sensitive and culturally informed interventions to address the disparities experienced by Santal women and promote gender equity within their patriarchal social structure.

Along with contributing to the existing theories, this study has addressed some of the methodological and conceptual gaps that exist in the literature as well. Most of the studies found on healthcare accessibility of poor people were quantitative research. Very few qualitative studies were found as well, but they were all secondary source-based and not empirical in nature. This study produces empirical evidence from firsthand field data. This in-depth empirical qualitative study will provide an extensive idea about the unequal access to healthcare services by ethnic women in Bangladesh. In the review of the literature, no study was found that takes into account the healthcare needs of ethnic women exclusively. Also, no study on the healthcare of Bangladeshi people has adopted an intersectional framework to take a better look at the healthcare needs and accessibility of disadvantaged rural women. Thus, methodology-wise, this study is a new addition to the existing body of knowledge.

Policy Suggestions

Through extensive field investigation, discernible impediments hindering healthcare accessibility have been unveiled, prompting the urgent need for apt policy interventions and the efficient execution of extant healthcare measures. Delving into the intricacies of these predicaments, the subsequent section offers insightful recommendations, aiming to bolster healthcare accessibility for marginalized Santal women. Moreover, it is evident that specific governmental health policies exhibit perplexing ambiguities regarding their approach to confronting the prevailing de facto disparities within the healthcare ecosystem. A resolute pursuit of equality and inclusivity in the healthcare domain necessitates meticulous explication and elucidation of these ambiguities to effectuate a transformative and equitable healthcare landscape.

The following steps can be taken to improve healthcare accessibility for ethnic women in Bangladesh:

1. The healthcare inclusivity index in Bangladesh lags behind that of most other Asian countries, indicating a need for enhanced focus in this area. Government documents inadequately prioritize inclusive healthcare, with policies often targeting the disadvantaged and poor population as a whole. While certain policies address the healthcare needs of ethnic groups in the Chittagong Hill Tracts (CHT), ethnic women, who constitute the primary recipients of health services at Universal Health Coverage facilities and are more susceptible to seeking maternal healthcare from these centers, do not receive specific attention. Additionally, ethnic communities residing on the mainland are not accounted for in policy documents, despite facing heightened public health challenges due to acute poverty, limited health literacy, lack of awareness, and constrained access to safe water and sanitation. To rectify these disparities, healthcare policies should be restructured to be inclusive and prioritize the health needs of ethnic women.

2. The healthcare accessibility of Santal women faces significant challenges primarily rooted in healthcare financing. The absence of institutional support and high out-of-pocket payments deter them from recognizing their healthcare needs. Moreover, the lack of suitable healthcare loan schemes by NGOs and non-profit organizations further exacerbates the situation. Additionally, the utilization of healthcare insurance remains unpopular among the Bangladeshi population, including ethnic groups. Although the Government of Bangladesh (GoB) is striving to achieve universal health coverage through initiatives like **Shastho Shurokkha Kormosuchi**, substantial progress in this regard is yet to be achieved. To enhance healthcare accessibility for rural ethnic women, introducing healthcare loans and insurance facilities specifically tailored for them could prove to be a viable solution.

3. Various efforts have been undertaken to enhance accessibility to information concerning public services and healthcare awareness. Nevertheless, the actual utilization of such information remains uncertain. For instance, the implementation of citizen charters enables individuals to become acquainted with the services available at public healthcare facilities. However, individuals with limited formal education do not derive substantial benefits from this information. Additionally, some health-related information is disseminated through websites, which ethnic women rarely access due to their limited knowledge and ownership of digital devices. Notably, during the COVID-19 pandemic, NGOs conducted awareness campaigns using billboard displays with health-related information conveyed through pictures. Such endeavors have proven valuable for individuals with little or no formal education. To ensure effective utilization of health information, dissemination strategies should take into account the educational levels of the target population. By doing so, these efforts can better reach and benefit those with limited educational backgrounds, promoting equitable access to healthcare knowledge.

4. The government should increase its healthcare budget allocation. A number of inefficiencies, such as an inadequate number of health providers, shortage of medicine, and poor quality of machines and services at the UHCs are a result of inadequate funds. Some of these issues are manageable at the local level through the funds of the UHCs, but others, like the appointment of health providers, are a concern of the central authority. Along with these, to ensure greater accountability in the health sector, reforms need to be introduced that will prevent the mismanagement of public funds.

5. Cooperation between government, non-government, and non-profit actors in the area of healthcare has been successful during the COVID-19 pandemic. This mighty pandemic has been fought and managed gracefully, with the minimum loss occurring in the study area. Thus, cooperative efforts by different actors to achieve common public health goals in the future can be a significant step toward efficient health management and public healthcare service delivery.

6. Discriminatory remarks and preferential treatment of the local elites by the NUHC health providers have discouraged Santal women from seeking healthcare from the NUHC. This is a serious issue and needs to be taken seriously. Policies can be made to educate health

providers on diversity and inclusion. The provision of punishment can be introduced and enforced strictly if evidence of discriminatory treatment and absenteeism by health providers is found.

SCOPE FOR FUTURE RESEARCH

This present study is focused on Santal women's healthcare access during the time of the COVID-19 pandemic outbreak. During that time, many factors of accessibility were hard to attain. For instance, imposed lockdowns and movement restrictions made transportation and mobility harder than in normal times. On top of that, the household income of Santals was also decreasing. The healthcare awareness of the Santal people has also increased during the pandemic outbreak, which has the potential to alter their health behavior significantly in the near future. Along with this, pandemic management and awareness-building efforts that have been proven successful during the coronavirus pandemic are worth exploring in detail to get better insights into their applicability and utility in future public health emergencies.

Another potential area for future research is the roles of NGOs, non-profits, and Christian missionaries in healthcare service delivery to the ethnic women of Bangladesh. Private healthcare facilities play a complementary role, along with public healthcare facilities, in delivering healthcare services to ethnic people. However, the extent and quality of these services are not properly explored in the scientific literature. Arguably, the monitoring mechanisms of private healthcare facilities are inefficient, along with their quality. So, the role of private healthcare facilities and the quality of private health services in Bangladesh require further exploration.

Lastly, this study has highlighted a number of challenges that create barriers for ethnic women (including Santal women) to access healthcare services. The ill-treatment by health providers and discriminatory attitudes toward ethnic women have been identified as two of the major factors. Educational attainment, although safeguarding ethnic men from such situations, isn't the case for Santal women. The limited scope of this study didn't allow the researcher to further explore this issue. This issue can be explored further in future research.

Conclusion

This chapter discusses the key findings of the study, their contribution to the current body of knowledge, and policy suggestions based on the field investigation of the study. There are a number of constitutional provisions, policies, programs, and projects run by the GoB to promote inclusive healthcare service delivery, ensure universal healthcare coverage, and provide equal healthcare to all. However, these policy documents and government plans and programs have remained inefficient to a great extent due to poor implementation of these policies. Government attempts have failed to increase the awareness of ethnic women and make healthcare more accessible to them. The issue of accessibility of healthcare for ethnic women thus needs to be considered in the healthcare policies. The government cannot achieve its goal of universal health coverage for all by 2032 leaving the Santal women behind both in policies and in practice.

References

Akter, S., Davies, K., Rich, J. L., & Inder, K. J. (2020). Barriers to accessing maternal health care services in the Chittagong Hill Tracts, Bangladesh: A qualitative descriptive study of Indigenous women's experiences. *PLoS ONE, 15*(8), e0237002. https://doi.org/10.1371/journal.pone.0237002

Ali, M. Y., Rahman, M. R., Javed, A., Toppo, A., & Akhtar, M. R. (2016). Indigenous Santal people sense and etiology regarding black fever illness. *American Journal of Health Research, 4*(5), 143.

Ame, A. S., Mozumdar, L., & Islam, M. A. (2021). Impact of social networks on the choice of place of delivery among ethnic women in Bangladesh. *Sexual & Reproductive Healthcare, 28*, 100588. https://doi.org/10.1016/j.srhc.2020.100588

Andersen, R. (1995). Revisiting the behavioral model and access to medical care: Does it matter? *Journal of Health and Social Behavior, 36*, 1–10.

Islam, M. R., & Odland, J. O. (2011). Determinants of antenatal and postnatal care visits among Indigenous people in Bangladesh: A study of the Mru community. *Rural Remote Health, 11*(2).

Khandakar, M. S. A. (2014). Rural health care system and patients' satisfaction towards medical care in Bangladesh: An empirical study. *Journal of Business Studies, 35*(2).

Levesque, J. F., Harris, M. F., & Russell, G. (2013). Patient-centered access to health care: Conceptualizing access at the interface of health systems and populations. *International Journal for Equity in Health, 12*(1).

Macdonald, G. (2021, February 4). *The challenges facing plainland ethnic groups in Bangladesh: Land, dignity, and inclusion.* International Republican Institute. Retrieved July 29, 2023, from https://www.iri.org/resources/new-bangladesh-report-examines-needs-of-plainland-ethnic-groups/

WHO. (2022, December 10). *Human rights.* Retrieved July 28, 2023, from https://shorturl.at/dvwAG

Index[1]

A

Access, v, vi, 2–6, 8, 9, 11, 12, 18–20, 26–27, 32, 33, 38–48, 51–69, 71, 72, 76, 77, 79, 81, 83, 84, 86–89, 93–105

Accessibility, 2–6, 11–13, 18–20, 26, 27, 34, 38, 39, 41, 44–47, 52, 58, 63, 68, 71, 73, 76, 78–81, 89, 90, 93, 94, 97–106

Affordability, 12, 39, 63, 68, 74, 79, 81, 83, 100

Antenatal, 30, 31, 45, 73

B

Bangladesh, v, 2–6, 8, 13, 15, 19, 20, 25–34, 38, 43–46, 51, 52, 54, 58, 59, 63, 66, 72, 76, 77, 79, 80, 85, 86, 89, 93, 98–100, 102, 103, 105

Behavioral change, 6, 61, 62

Birth attendant, 31

C

Chapainawabganj, 4, 13, 16

Chittagong Hill Tract (CHT), 27, 44, 63, 99, 103

Community, v, 3, 8–10, 13, 17, 27, 28, 31, 33, 40, 44–48, 52, 54–56, 59–61, 63, 65–68, 77, 79, 82–84, 89, 93–99, 101–103

Contraceptives, 8, 31, 58

Cooperative, 68, 69, 81, 82, 96, 104

Costs, 33, 45, 54–57, 78–81, 83, 84, 97

COVID-19, v, vi, 2–10, 15, 18–20, 27, 32, 33, 38, 47, 51, 52, 54, 56, 58–68, 72, 74, 77–81, 84, 86–89, 95, 96, 101, 104, 105

Credit, 82, 83

D

DASCOH Foundation, 64, 65, 67, 82

Decision-making, 72, 80, 94

[1] Note: Page numbers followed by 'n' refer to notes.

© The Author(s), under exclusive license to Springer Nature Switzerland AG 2023
F. Nawaz, AN Bushra, *Santal Women and the Health Care Regime*,
https://doi.org/10.1007/978-3-031-48872-6

Doctor, 31, 34, 54, 56, 57, 73,
    75–77, 80, 81, 84, 85, 88, 97

E
Education, 2, 6, 7, 9, 26, 30, 31, 33,
    45, 46, 57–61, 63, 68, 74,
    95, 99, 104
Employment, 43, 44, 72
Empower, 6, 48
Equal healthcare, 2, 3, 7, 19,
    25, 44, 106
Equitable healthcare, vi, 2, 6, 26, 33,
    38, 40, 94, 97, 103, 104
Ethnicity, v, vi, 13, 14, 30, 42, 43,
    55–58, 98, 100, 101
Ethnic women, 2, 9, 13, 16, 18–20,
    32, 38–48, 52, 55, 93, 94,
    98–100, 102–106

F
Family planning, 5, 30
Financial status, 78–80

G
Gender, v, vi, 6–8, 13, 14, 19, 26, 30,
    38, 39, 41–45, 42n1, 47, 52,
    54–58, 60, 78, 86, 89, 93,
    94, 98–102
Government of Bangladesh (GoB), 19,
    25–27, 31, 32, 34, 54, 66,
    103, 106

H
Healthcare budget, 32, 99, 104
Healthcare cost, 56, 79–81, 83
Healthcare financing, 78, 81–83, 103
Healthcare policy, 2, 19, 26, 94,
    103, 106

Healthcare providers, 30–32, 34
Healthcare seeking, 63, 95, 100, 101
Healthcare utilization, 38, 40–42, 100
Health literacy, 44–46, 59–61,
    86, 89, 103
Health providers, 16, 18, 20, 41,
    54–58, 71–77, 85, 87–90, 97, 98,
    100, 101, 104, 105
Health-related information,
    44, 67, 104
Health-seeking behavior, 15, 19, 20,
    40, 44, 47, 54, 60, 63, 75, 84,
    100, 101
Hospital, 4, 5, 10, 28, 31, 33, 34, 53,
    56, 57, 72, 76, 80, 82, 84,
    86, 88, 97

I
Identity marker, 6, 9
Inclusive, vi, 6, 27, 43, 98, 103, 106
Inclusivity, 25–34, 73–75, 97, 98, 103
Income, 2, 33, 59, 62, 78–81,
    78n1, 105
Indigenous, v, 8, 31, 44–46,
    59, 73, 84
Inequality, v, 3, 5–9, 26, 38, 41, 42,
    47, 51, 58, 79, 98, 102
Institution, 5, 10, 11, 14, 31, 34, 54,
    58, 63, 82, 83, 95, 100
Intersectional approach, 3, 8
Intersectionality, 8, 38, 41–44, 101

L
Literacy, 59, 63, 68, 87–89, 95, 96, 102
Local, 5, 13, 16, 17, 28, 40, 57, 58,
    65, 67, 68, 73, 77, 78, 83, 96, 104
Local level, 15, 19, 28, 30, 32,
    40, 45, 104
Lockdown, 3–5, 33, 59, 60, 78,
    79, 88, 105

M
Marginalization, 6, 32, 42, 43, 84
Marginalized, v, 6, 8, 26, 27, 31, 40,
    42, 44, 48, 84, 96, 97, 100, 102
Medical care, 2, 26, 86
Mismanagement, 5, 33, 99, 104
Missionary, 31, 82, 105
Mobility, 56, 78, 100, 105

N
Nachol, 77, 82, 88
Nachol Upazila Health Complex
    (NUHC), 54–58, 61, 63–65, 67,
    68, 71–77, 86–89, 96, 97,
    101, 104
Non-ethnic women, 17, 18, 20, 52,
    55, 60, 61, 66, 68, 72, 73, 75,
    79, 82, 87, 95, 96, 101
Non-profit, 10, 30, 89, 103–105

P
Pandemic, v, vi, 2–9, 18–20, 38, 42,
    43, 47, 51–54, 58, 59, 61–63,
    66, 68, 69, 71–90, 95, 96, 101,
    102, 104, 105
Policy, 2, 6, 19, 20, 26–28, 32, 40, 42,
    47, 48, 63, 93, 94, 98, 102–106
Politicians, 13, 17, 57, 83
Postnatal, 30, 31, 45, 73
Power, 16, 40, 47, 89
Pregnancy, 8, 45, 55, 80
Preventive, 26, 31
Private healthcare, 10, 30–32, 53–56,
    63, 64, 95, 97, 100, 101, 105
Public health, 2, 4, 5, 9–11, 26, 27,
    32, 33, 44, 47, 54, 63, 68, 69,
    93, 94, 96, 99, 103–105
Public healthcare, 2, 5, 9–12, 16, 18,
    26, 30, 32–34, 46, 47, 53, 54, 58,
    68, 76–78, 94, 95, 99, 104, 105

Public service, 5, 6, 38, 104

Q
Qualitative data, 16, 18
Qualitative research, 13, 47, 99
Quantitative research, 94, 99, 102

R
Reproductive health, 31, 32, 47

S
Santal women, v, vi, 2, 6, 15–20, 38,
    44, 47, 51–69, 71–90,
    94–98, 100–106
Service providers, 10–12
Service recipients, 5–6, 11, 12, 38, 39,
    41, 58, 74, 76
Social identity, 40, 42, 83, 94, 100
Social structure, 40, 52, 101–102
Socio-economic status, 13, 18, 43, 45,
    68, 94, 98

T
Theoretical Framework, 8, 38
Traditional, v, 31, 45, 46, 84,
    85, 96, 97
Transportation, 45, 47, 55, 58, 81,
    83, 100, 105
Treatment, 5, 8–11, 33, 45, 46,
    54–58, 60–63, 72, 73, 80, 82–85,
    89, 95, 97, 100, 101, 104, 105
Tribal, 52, 54
Trust, 53, 54, 58–61, 76, 95

U
Union, 5, 28
Universal health coverage, 27, 103, 106

Upazila, 27
Upazila Health Complex(UHC),
    5, 18, 28, 30, 47, 52–54,
    56–58, 71–77, 80, 81, 83,
    95, 101, 104
Utilization, 11, 26, 38,
    40–42, 45, 53, 97, 100,
    101, 103, 104

V
Vaccination, 10, 33, 57, 58, 60, 61,
    63–68, 73, 95, 96
Vaccine, 4, 7, 32, 57, 65–67

W
Well-being, 2, 9, 11, 27